The Journey to Parenthood

Myths, reality and what really matters

Diana Lynn Barnes, Psy.D.
and
Leigh G. Balber

Foreword by

Roberta Michnick Golinkoff
and
Kathy Hirsh-Pasek

Radcliffe Publishing
Oxford • New York

Radcliffe Publishing Ltd
18 Marcham Road
Abingdon
Oxon OX14 1AA
United Kingdom

www.radcliffe-oxford.com
Electronic catalogue and worldwide online ordering facility.

British Library Cataloguing in Publication Data

A catalogue record for this book is available from the British Library.

ISBN-10 1 84619 014 2
ISBN-13 978 1 84619 014 8

Typeset by Ann Buchan (Typesetters), Middlesex, UK
Printed and bound by T J I Digital Ltd, Padstow, Cornwall, UK

Contents

To my daughter, Danielle – your birth and loving presence in my life have opened the door to a most remarkable journey. (D.L.B.)

To Scott and Emma – who light the way with laughter and love. (L.G.B.)

Foreword

One morning, Roberta was waiting patiently for a photographer to arrive to take her picture for a magazine article. The photographer, Sarah, was already 15 minutes late. And then, as if on cue, there was a flurry of knocks at the door and Sarah rushed in, apologizing profusely for her tardiness. She had a great excuse: She was a brand-new mom, and it had taken longer than she had anticipated to drop off her child at daycare on her way to the appointment. As new parents will come to learn, getting a baby ready to go somewhere is a lot like flying on any one of the schedule-challenged airlines, with unexpected delays and a very loose definition of the phrase "on time."

When Roberta told Sarah how fabulous it was that she had just delivered a healthy, 8-pound baby boy, Sarah admitted that she was very excited to photograph Roberta because – as she said in a breathy and slightly panicked voice – she wanted to ask her when to introduce her young son to flash cards. The irony was that Sarah had come to photograph Roberta for our latest book entitled *Einstein Never Used Flash Cards: How Our Children Really Learn and Why They Need to Play More and Memorize Less*! But Sarah, in her new mom haze, either hadn't read the title or had misinterpreted it. She seemed genuinely alarmed about failing her 6-week-old baby because she hadn't yet started his intellectual training.

This is not an unusual story. And the parenting hype begins long before a baby ever sets eyes on his first pile of flash cards. It is now so ingrained in our culture that it is as much a part of the journey to parenthood as is the awe of seeing that first ultrasound. This "cult of achievement" has added a whole new level of anxiety for expectant mothers and fathers. As a result, they feel pressure to accomplish a set of goals that has nothing to do with the more important process of becoming a parent.

Mothers-to-be tend to obsess about maintaining their pre-pregnancy figures. They believe that having an epidural is a sign of weakness, indicative of some sort of character flaw. Men who take on duties in the delivery room assume they have disappointed their wives if they are unable to anticipate their every need or fail to provide the physical comfort their wives so desperately want. In addition, new mothers and fathers fault themselves for not immediately knowing how to calm their crying babies or get them to sleep for a period of longer than 20 minutes. And then there are the pressures both expectant and new parents feel to spend their hard-earned dollars on questionable goods and services – electronic "educational" toys, French lessons for babies and, yes, flash cards – in an effort to boost their little ones' intelligence.

The Journey to Parenthood is the antidote to this culture's insanity about preparing for parenthood. In these pages, you will learn that there is no such thing as the "perfect parent," and that when parents follow their instincts, they are probably doing the best thing possible to be good parents, and to raise intelligent and happy babies. You will also learn that getting ready to become a mother or father is about contemplating what kind of parent one would like to be. It is about considering how parenthood might affect one's career, marriage and priorities, even one's day-to-day routine.

We suggest future and new parents follow the mantra, "reflect, resist and re-center" that we introduce in *Einstein*. Expectant parents need to *reflect* on what they have heard in the media – and from their Aunt Ida – about parenting and what their new roles will entail. They should *resist* the urge to be swept away by the parenting hype and instead stay attuned to their own thoughts, feelings and experiences as they become parents. And finally, they need to *re-center*, to reassure themselves they have made good choices based on their own ideas and values. In *Einstein Never Used Flash Cards*, we point out how "childhood is about making discoveries." So too is the journey to parenthood.

Roberta Michnick Golinkoff and Kathy Hirsh-Pasek,
Authors of *Einstein Never Used Flash Cards: How Our Children*
Really Learn and Why They Need to Play More and Memorize Less
January 2007

Preface

I gave birth to my daughter 14 years ago. Back then it never occurred to me that what I had thought was supposed to be a time of ultimate fulfillment would become a life-threatening crisis. I had always dreamed of raising a girl. After giving birth to a son 11 years earlier, I was finally going to get that chance. Despite a difficult pregnancy marked by severe dehydration that landed me in the hospital, toxemia, and my husband's heart attack two weeks before the birth, nothing could mar the wonderful mother–daughter images I envisioned of special lunch dates, shopping, sharing clothes and secrets. Given how much I had come to embrace the pregnancy, what followed came as a complete shock.

After my daughter was born, I felt confused, withdrawn and hopeless. I lived in a disoriented state, and my memory was hazy. Any confidence I had developed regarding my competency as a mother was eroded by panic and by growing feelings of inadequacy. I longed to care for my infant daughter and to cradle her in my arms, but I was paralyzed by anxiety. I was overwhelmed by the mere thought of having to take care of her, and then felt guilty because, after all, I had desperately wanted her. And so what I had hoped would be a blossoming relationship was disrupted by this relentless nightmare. The constant struggle against suicidal impulses overpowered me until one year and four hospitalizations later, when doctors finally gave my illness a name – postpartum depression.

My arduous uphill battle toward recovery led me to discover that I was not alone in having this illness. Between 10% and 20% of women who give birth will suffer from some form of a postpartum mood disorder. It is not necessary for a woman to wait until the postpartum period to find out whether she will be in that group. Pregnancy is the perfect time for her, along with her partner, to assess her risks and to devise a strategy for minimizing stress during the transition to parenthood.

For the past decade, I have been exploring the emotional journey to parenthood with expectant parents who attend my *Transition to Parenthood* workshops in the Los Angeles area. Most of the mothers- and fathers-to-be who participate in the workshops welcome the opportunity to talk about themselves and their expectations regarding childbirth and the journey to parenthood. These are not topics they typically have an opportunity to discuss during other prenatal classes or at their regular appointments with their obstetricians.

The hundreds of couples – from a wide range of socio-economic and ethnic backgrounds – who have shared their thoughts with me about becoming parents, as well as my own battle with postpartum depression and my personal experience as a parent, all inspired me to write this book.

Diana Lynn Barnes
Center for Postpartum Health
Woodland Hills, CA
January 2007

About the authors

Diana Lynn Barnes, Psy.D., MFT, an internationally recognized expert in the field of perinatal mood disorders, is a psychotherapist who has been writing and speaking on family issues and women's mental health for over 20 years. She is the author of *Celebrity Parenting: famous parents share personal stories* and the creator/producer of *The Parent Profile*, a CBS nationally syndicated radio feature. In addition to her private practice, she teaches Family Studies and Child Development at Los Angeles Valley College and Pierce College. The past president of Postpartum Support International, Diana created and teaches a monthly seminar for expectant parents called *Transition to Parenthood*. She lives in Los Angeles with her son and daughter.

Leigh G. Balber is a freelance writer whose work has appeared in *Child* magazine, *American Baby* magazine and on BabyZone.com. She spent a decade in television news, writing and producing for CBS News, CNBC TV and Court TV. She lives in New York City with her husband and daughter.

Acknowledgements

Not unlike pregnancy and childbirth, the birth of a book involves a gestational period of its own. After an idea is conceived, it can only become a book after months and months of meticulous planning and preparation. With the support of a number of very special people, this book – *The Journey to Parenthood: Myths, Reality and What Really Matters* – was born.

Our heartfelt thanks go to Gillian Nineham and the editors at Radcliffe who saw the wisdom in this book and supported us in bringing the manuscript to life.

We offer our deepest thanks to Emily Haverstick, who helped to nurture this project by spending hundreds of hours compiling research. In addition, Caroline Elman, Linda Folse, Juanita Sanchez and Stacy Simone, the librarians at Phillips Graduate Institute in Los Angeles, worked laboriously to deliver research materials at a moment's notice. Thank you, Scott Balber, for tirelessly reading and re-reading copy, long after your own business day was done. We are extremely grateful to our assistant, Candyce Carpenter, who kept us organized by always managing to stay one step ahead of us.

Obstetrician/gynecologist Dr. Rebecca Perlow honored us as a consultant, in order to ensure that this book would be medically accurate and current. Thank you, Elaine Hanzak, our friend across the ocean, who through a twist of fate brought us together with Radcliffe. Wendy Kelman directs the Women's Resource Center and prenatal education classes at Tarzana Hospital in Tarzana, California. Recognizing how essential it is for expectant parents to understand the psychological impact of the pregnancy experience, she provided a home for the *Transition to Parenthood* workshop, which formed the basis for this book. We would also like to thank pediatrician Lynn Osher, Dr. Alison Zimon, who is a reproductive endocrinologist with Boston IVF and Beth Israel Deaconess Medical Center and who is also a clinical instructor at Harvard Medical School, Dr. Peter Schmidt, Chief of the Unit on Reproductive Endocrinology at the Behavioral Endocrinology Branch of the National Institute of Mental Health, Ellen Galinsky, who runs the Families and Work Institute in New York, Teresa Hamdan, Julie Balber, Pamela Madsen with the American Fertility Association, Eleanor Nicoll with the American Society for Reproductive Medicine, Mocha Moms, the Woman's Hospital in Baton Rouge, Louisiana, and the MacDonald Women's Hospital of University Hospitals of Cleveland.

Of course, this book could never have been written without the wonderful couples who welcomed us into their lives. They shared their most private thoughts and feelings so that other expectant parents might realize the importance of exploring their own emotional experiences as they make the journey to parenthood.

Introduction

First-time parents are a gullible group that just loves guarantees. They will read any book that promises perfect parenting by the final chapter. They will buy any musical mobile that has been billed as a surefire way to boost a baby's IQ. Pregnant women flock to childbirth classes with instructors who swear that their approaches to labor and delivery will lead to relaxing, pain-free experiences on the big day.

Insecure about assuming such a significant role, which is like nothing they have ever done before, expectant parents are willing to do whatever it takes to make certain they get the right start on the parenting track. But preparing for parenthood is not just about doing or buying. It is about contemplating what it really means to be a parent. It is about recognizing how a baby will irrevocably transform their lives as individuals and as a couple.

In addition to focusing on guarantees, expectant parents also tend to pay close attention to the physical aspects of pregnancy – the weight gain, the diagnostic tests, the ultrasounds, the lists of foods a mother should and should not eat. Although these are all significant and deserving of attention, most people do not take stock of how they feel about impending parenthood and all that their new roles will entail. The journey to parenthood is far more complex than many realize. Typically, most parents-to-be understand that a new little person in their lives will mean *some* additional work, but they have no idea just how much. Nor can most expectant couples anticipate the many ways in which becoming a parent will change their identities, their priorities and the daily rhythms of their lives forever.

We live in a society that glorifies pregnancy and parenthood. A new life is certainly worth celebrating, but many men and women muddle through this enormous transition feeling inadequate, scared, stressed and even angry. In some ways, new parents have been set up to fail by cultural ideals that characterize the birth of a child as the most wonderful time in a couple's life. Society has sugar-coated the realities of the first-time parenting experience, leaving many new parents with a saccharine aftertaste. As a result, these new parent initiates believe they are not experiencing the real thing but some mediocre substitute, when they do not feel an instant bond with their babies, when they do not sense a more intense love in their marriages, and when the postpartum period does not consist of endless joy but rather of tension, unpredictability and a yearning for the way life used to be.

This book attempts to debunk some of the myths about pregnancy and parenting while offering readers a glimpse into the lives and minds of first-time parents, both before and after delivery. These mothers and fathers, who come from a wide range of socio-economic and ethnic backgrounds, compare their expectations with the realities of pregnancy, labor and delivery, and the postpartum period. They discuss how they came to form their various beliefs about childbirth and the transition to parenthood, and how those expectations affected their adjustment to family life.

By exploring the psychological side of pregnancy and new parenthood, mothers- and fathers-to-be can start to identify, discuss and address concerns before the baby arrives. They can begin to pinpoint, and maybe even alleviate, certain stresses prior to the postpartum period, when new parents must contend with sleepless nights and the new baby learning curve. Exploration questions are included at the end of the book so that couples can start to contemplate and discuss their own thoughts and feelings about impending parenthood.

Chapter 1 identifies those myths we hear about, and come to accept as true, on the journey to parenthood. Because the physiological aspects of pregnancy – what we can see, measure and physically feel – are such an obvious and integral part of bringing a new baby into the world, an entire chapter – Chapter 2 – is devoted to the mind–body connection of pregnancy. The physical changes in the woman's body can trigger the beginning of an emotional tie between both parents and their unborn baby. But the pregnancy transformation can also affect a woman's body image, as well as feelings about sexual intimacy.

This book also examines how expectant and new parents define their own parenting styles and what it means to be a "good father" and a "good mother." It looks at the transition to parenthood from three distinct perspectives – that of the woman, the man and the couple. Chapter 3 delves into the psychological experience of motherhood, Chapter 4, the psychological experience of fatherhood and, later in the book, Chapter 7 explores the couple's changing relationship. It is important to understand the unique viewpoints men and women bring to parenting, and how they mesh their separate ideas and opinions to form a collective parenting unit.

Chapter 5 breaks down the labor and delivery experience. It analyzes women's expectations regarding pain, the length and difficulty of the childbirth process, and their partners' abilities to comfort and assist them. Chapter 5 also looks at men's expectations concerning their roles in the delivery room. In addition, couples share their reactions to what is supposed to be the most dramatic and emotional event of the whole nine months: the baby's debut.

Welcoming a baby into the family and into the home is often nothing short of chaotic. In Chapter 6, new parents talk about what life is like once they bring their babies home from the hospital. They discuss their frustrations in trying to figure out just what their babies need, why they might be crying and why they are not sleeping "like babies." The chapter addresses the conflicts that can arise when a new division of labor is required to accommodate all of the additional work in the postpartum period. It also offers some practical advice on what parents can do about the hordes of new baby well-wishers who visit or phone. With good intentions, these friends, colleagues and family members often have a tendency to dispense advice on anything and everything having to do with babies. They inundate the rookie moms and dads with suggestions on how to feed, clothe, diaper, swaddle, soothe, rock, bathe and dress a baby. However, at such a pivotal juncture in the transition to parenthood, this advice can undermine new parents because this is the time when they are just getting to know their infant and just beginning to gain confidence in their parenting abilities.

Chapter 8 presents an overview of postpartum depression and other perinatal mood illnesses, their causes, symptoms and treatments. The chapter identifies which women have a greater risk of developing a mood disorder in the period surrounding childbirth, and it recommends certain measures women (as well as men) can take during pregnancy to try to prevent the onset of depression, or at least lessen the severity of the symptoms. Approximately 13% of women who have babies will develop some form of postpartum depression.

And finally, because there are so many different ways to put together a family today, and because modern medicine has provided us with the technology to help people create babies, Chapter 9 looks at the many paths to parenthood and variations on the traditional family. It explains the unique issues and conditions that define those mothers' and fathers' journeys to parenthood.

Thinking about the psychological experience of becoming a parent, and identifying and managing certain fears and sources of potential conflict, can make the transition to parenthood smoother, giving parents a sense of order amidst the turmoil of the hectic postpartum period. This psychological dress rehearsal does not guarantee a seamless shift from couple to family, but it can decrease the likelihood that these issues will take center stage once the baby is born. As the curtain rises on this new chapter in a couple's life, they will want to do everything possible to enjoy the show.

CHAPTER 1

Beginning the journey

The most important job is that of a parent, for a parent is completely responsible for the life of another person. A mother and father must ensure the survival of a tiny human being who needs help eating, falling asleep, staying clean and staying happy. A parent is charged with the awesome and, at first, seemingly incomprehensible mission of taking a seven-pound infant who cannot even hold up her (or his) head, caring for her, and then guiding her through the years into adulthood, when she herself becomes an independent, contributing member of society.

As new parents fulfill their infant's basic needs for food, comfort and love, they get to know her by learning to decode her unique communication signals, determining whether the distinctive pitches of her cries indicate that she is hungry, tired or just in need of being cuddled. Later, they will teach this new little person how to walk, talk, feed and bathe herself. They will also teach her how to share with others, function within a group and achieve her personal goals. And most likely it is a child's parents who will eventually show her how to deal with failure, success, heartbreak and life's countless dilemmas along the way. When two people resolve to have children, they are making a lifelong commitment to travel a road that will be paved with magical moments, mistakes and, sometimes, unbelievable frustration. But through all of this, they will come to know a love like no other.

Strange as it may sound, the process of becoming a parent begins long before the birth of a child. Throughout our lives, we take "mental snapshots" of parenthood. Even as young children, our brains record how responsive our parents are to our needs and demands, and how affectionate or loving they are when we are in distress. We arrange these pictures into a sort of psychological scrapbook, identifying what we like, what has been helpful for us and what has made us feel special, but also what has made us feel sad, mad or unloved. We carry these mental images of our relationships with our parents into adulthood and then use them to help determine what kind of parents we would like to be. They help us decide what we will repeat and what we will do differently when it is our turn to parent.

As young children, we begin to model what we observe of parenthood not only in our own homes, but also in the homes of our friends and relatives. And we take cues about what it means to be a parent from the news media, as well as from fictional characters portrayed on television and in the movies. As we get older, we are better able to crystallize these memories and observations. For example, a woman may readily recall the first time she was punished for slapping her little sister, or a special pizza dinner out with mom to celebrate nothing more than the end of a particularly bad day. All of this becomes the foundation for parenthood.

The decision to start a family may depend upon any number of factors. Many of the couples interviewed for this book cited age, financial comfort and job stability among their main reasons for choosing to have a baby. Thirty-four-year-old Jennifer, a mother of twins, notes that she was one of those women who worried about the ticking of the proverbial biological clock. The Dallas mom says she thought to herself, "We're older, so we'd better start trying because who knows how long it will take. A lot of my friends had trouble, trouble, trouble."

Regarding his decision to have kids, Ralph, a radio manager, says, "I was 34 when we were married. I was financially stable. It was something that I had always wanted to do. I think a lot of people say, 'We don't want to have kids yet because we want to travel or we want to live in this big house first or we need to remodel the kitchen,' those kinds of things. I think our lives were pretty fulfilled at that point so we were ready to take that step."

Roberto,* originally from Venezuela, is now a marketing sales director with a cosmetics company in Los Angeles. He recalls, "Starting two years ago, my wife and I got everything into place because, at first, we didn't have any stability at all. And, of course, if you don't have stability, I don't think you should consider having a child." He describes their previous financial circumstances, "We were living in a one-bedroom apartment. I lost my job, she lost her job, we lived on credit cards." Eventually, they both found work. "And then somehow we got the house and from there it was time," says Roberto.

Roberto also says his desire to have a child was part of a deeper need for a fulfillment that could not be realized through financial or career accomplishments. "I got to the point where I had achieved what society tells you that you need to achieve, and then there was some kind of emptiness, especially being in L.A. where there's this culture of 'me, me, me.' And then you get tired of that because how can you only be obsessed with yourself?"

While some people consider the decision to start a family a simple and obvious one, others, like Roberto's wife, Kelly, contend that it is not so straightforward. She had mixed feelings about bringing a child into her world. Three-and-a-half months before her daughter, Emma, was born, Kelly said, "I'm scared about it. I have all these emotions I'm dealing with. I feel trapped on one level because I've always been pretty independent. I feel ecstatic on another level. We just did the hospital tour and when I saw those little babies, I felt all emotional and started crying." Kelly, who used to run an independent film production company, continues, "Part of me is just really terrified. I know

---

*Some names have been changed at the request of interviewees.

it's not going to be about me anymore. I'm used to having my freedom, living my life ... I don't see myself as a stay-at-home mom 24 hours a day. I think I'd kill myself. But I love the baby, I feel her, I'm excited to have her. I'll do the best that I can do."

Jim and Janine, transplanted Minnesotans who moved to New York, were ready to settle down and start a family after enjoying their life as a couple and taking what they called their "lifetime trips" to see the *Tour de France*, Italy, Alaska and Hawaii. Janine, like Jennifer, was also concerned about the age factor. She and Jim are both in their mid-30s. "That age thing was always in the back of my mind. The older I got, the harder it might be," she says. Both previously divorced, neither Jim nor Janine had wanted children before they met each other. Jim had a particularly traumatic childhood. He and his siblings lived in extreme poverty, surviving on welfare, food stamps and pinto beans. "My mom would soak pinto beans in a Crock-Pot and that would be our dinner for a week," he recalls. They moved around frequently, calling Indiana, Rhode Island, Nova Scotia and Texas "home" at one time or another. Jim says his mother and her second husband physically and verbally abused him, his brother and sister. After they were divorced, his mother wandered from boyfriend to boyfriend. Jim says that in addition to these hardships, his mother was an alcoholic and suffered from bipolar disorder, which went untreated until he was 14 years old.

"Having grown up in a pretty tough household – it was certainly not the most ideal of upbringings – I really had the feeling that with so many kids out there who need a good home, who don't have a stable household, and who really don't have the opportunity to go to good schools, why bring another child into the world? There are so many other needy kids out there. That was my mentality for a few years," explains Jim, continuing, "But when I met Janine, the tables turned on me, and I couldn't imagine not sharing the love we had in our lives with our own child." Janine emphasizes, "I felt like having a kid would complete our relationship and our life."

Thirty-six-year-old Tim thought of time in different terms than Janine and Jennifer did, citing his own inevitable mortality as the reason he hoped to start a family with his wife LeeRan while they were still relatively young. He wanted to make sure that he would be able to watch his children grow and develop and "still be alive, hopefully" when they became adults.

For Kate and Paul from Devon, England, the decision to start a family did not mean that they would begin "trying" to have a baby. Kate did not want to approach the act of creating a new life as a carefully planned, orchestrated event, but rather as something that would happen naturally, as an extension of their love for each other. "I don't want to have sex with my husband because I'm trying to have a child. I want to have sex with my husband because he's gorgeous, you know?" she giggles. She explains that when a couple focuses on trying to "make a baby," they exert undue pressure on themselves. "It takes something away from your sex life," she notes.

Sometimes starting a family requires no decision. It just happens. Two of the couples we interviewed had unplanned pregnancies. But for them, unplanned did not mean unwanted, even for Megan, a new mom from Missouri who was only 15 years old when she became pregnant. Before the pregnancy, Megan had never envisioned having a baby that young. That was supposed to come later, "in her 20s, at least." Megan's first reaction upon discovering that she was pregnant was: "Oh no ... I was thinking about whether I was going to finish school and if my mom was going to be mad at me." Megan's mother, Pam, had herself been a teenage mom. "I didn't want Megan to go through what I did being a teen mother," remarks Pam, adding that she used to tell her daughter, "'If you get pregnant, we're not having the baby.' And then as soon as I found out she was pregnant, that was no longer an issue." Pam said to her daughter, "The only thing I'm going to require is that you have to walk across the stage. You have to graduate." Megan did graduate and is now studying criminal justice at a local college. She ended up marrying the baby's father. Even though the pregnancy was unexpected, Megan embraced it. "I was actually really happy. I liked it. I liked the feeling that I was going to be bringing somebody else into the world."

Nakisha and Randall had a honeymoon baby. "We got married in July and we went to Hawaii for our honeymoon. In August, I didn't get my period, so I checked to see what was going on," recalls Nakisha, laughing. Sure enough, she was pregnant. As to the timing of the pregnancy, she says, "We never even really talked about how long we wanted to wait for kids. I mean I was ready in the sense that all the things that I needed, that I wanted in place beforehand, such as being married" and having a career, were set. Nakisha, who works in the Public Defender's Office in Washington, D.C., says that when she was a child, her plan was to have two kids by the time she was 30. So she is still on track to accomplish that goal.

Many of the parents interviewed said they had always wanted children. Others admitted that starting a family was not something they ever previously desired. Keri, a Kentucky mother working at a pharmaceutical company in research and development, comments, "When my husband and I got married, he wanted children, and I told him that if we never had children, I would be fine." It is not that she was opposed to having kids, just that she thought she could be satisfied without them. When Keri was 12 years old, she watched how motherhood affected her then 16-year-old sister. "I think that just kind of turned me off on having children, just seeing her struggle and the things that she had to do at the age of 16." But Keri says her husband, D.J., longed to have kids, "So it really wasn't an option not to have them."

D.J. happily credits their dog, Deke, with Keri's change of heart. "When we were dating, she was never a dog person and never really a kid person, and I talked her into getting a dog. That required every ounce of salesmanship I had. But we got a dog and instantly her heart melted for him ... I think having him in the house really brought out a lot of her maternal instincts," says D.J., an advertising sales manager at a major newspaper. He and Keri consider Deke to be a full-fledged member of the family – his name is even on the outgoing message of their answering-machine!

Neil will turn 50 just before his first child is born. When he and Robin got married, he was not sure whether he wanted to have children. "It was still a struggle for me to determine, 'Yes, I really want to go forward with this, or maybe this isn't right for me.'" Of his eventual decision to have a child, he says, "I knew it was important to my wife. We talked about what it would be like without a child. I just came to the realization that this was something that I was able to do. And probably if Robin hadn't wanted children, I wouldn't have been the one to say, 'Let's have a child.'" Neil concludes, "I think my love for Robin and the fact that I wanted our relationship to continue were big factors in my decision ... and ironically now we're thinking we have to have at least two children." He is quick to add that Robin never pressured him to start a family. "I think she knows that my personality is that if you push me, if you pressure me, I'm going to go the other way."

Neil explains his initial reluctance to have children: "I think that the whole process of having children and being a parent is glorified. Everybody says, 'Oh, it changes your life forever and for the better.' And I suppose overall it can, but there are a lot of issues that people just gloss over or deny or ignore – the fact that your freedom is cut dramatically, that a lot of things that you used to enjoy doing you either can't do as often or you can't do at all."

What Neil refers to as society's glorification of parenthood is a premise central to many of the myths about parenthood. These myths are predicated on the idea that having a child automatically enhances every aspect of one's life, and that being a parent is natural and automatic for everyone. Although the instinct to care for and protect one's children is inherent, many people need time and some hands-on training before parenthood feels a little more comfortable.

Facts, fiction and fantasy: the myths of parenting

Babies may embody all of the magic, innocence and wonderment of a fairy tale. But the realities of pregnancy, childbirth and the postpartum period can be a very different story. Illusions about the birth of a baby leave many expectant and new parents feeling ill-suited to the task of parenting. These rookie parents may be very accomplished in their chosen professions, running a division of a company, saving people's lives, defending the rights of those charged with a crime, or designing advertising campaigns for a Fortune 500 company. But when it comes to parenting, they often do not have the confidence they have acquired in other areas of their lives. This lack of confidence arises, in part, because of the societal myths we perpetuate. When new parents fail to meet the lofty expectations created by these myths, they may feel as if they have somehow been undermined, since no one told them what new parenthood was really like. Romantic ideals clash with reality at one of the most stressful and anxious times in the family life cycle, a time that researchers once labeled a "crisis" period. (More recently researchers have described this time period as a developmental transition in the life of a family.[1-4]) We are not conditioned to think of a new baby as anything other than blissful.

MYTH #1: All women "glow" during pregnancy

Of course, there are women who do glow during pregnancy. Their faces radiate contentment, they are flush with happiness, even their hair shines. For them, carrying a child is pure joy. It is almost as if we can picture them in some old-fashioned Broadway musical, breaking into a cheery song-and-dance number in the middle of the street, surrounded by the non-glowing, non-pregnant masses.

But not all women, or men for that matter, find this time in their lives pleasant or enjoyable. And because this lack of enthusiasm conflicts with what they have been led to believe about pregnancy, they can end up feeling unsure of themselves, questioning both their commitment to raising a child and their competence as parents. In silent guilt, they may ask themselves, "What's wrong with me? Why am I not ecstatic about this pregnancy?"

The reality is that many pregnancies are complicated and/or especially trying, and a difficult pregnancy can diminish or even extinguish "the glow." Also, an unplanned pregnancy, memories of an unhappy childhood, a bad relationship with one's own parents, a strained marriage, financial stresses, and concerns about balancing the various roles of spouse, parent and employee (or boss) can all weigh heavily as women and men adjust to the parenthood transition.

Traditionally, the focus during and immediately after pregnancy has been on physical matters – changes in the woman's body, the health of the mother and baby, and the mother's recovery. A mother's psychological well-being has been largely ignored. Although the physical aspects of pregnancy and childbirth deserve careful attention, it is also essential to consider the emotional states of both the mother and the father.

It is not likely that Jennifer would have described herself as glowing during pregnancy. "I had all these negative thoughts and feelings because people don't share the hard stuff," says the Dallas mother of twins. "People don't share the real scoop – that you're gassy, that you're hateful and that you don't want your husband to touch you. Nobody shares all of that fun pregnancy stuff. You get hair where you shouldn't be getting it. Your hair falls out. My hairline receded. Nobody told me about that. Everyone said, 'Your hair is going to get thick.' Well, my hair's naturally thick and shiny, and it got ugly."

Exuding "The Glow" is certainly not a prerequisite for becoming a good parent. It is understandable and perfectly normal for women to struggle with some of the discomforts of pregnancy and to worry about the new responsibilities they are about to assume. Discontentment with gas and ugly hair does not mean that a woman will be a bad mother or that her child will never go to college. Nor does it indicate an inability to love and care for a baby. In fact, being able to share one's feelings about pregnancy, and to talk about why it might not be the wonderful experience she had anticipated, can be liberating. A woman may feel a tremendous sense of relief after struggling alone with these thoughts and feelings. Discussing them with her husband, friend, doctor or another expectant mother may help relieve the guilt that has prevented her from enjoying her pregnancy and impending motherhood. This discussion provides the expectant mother with an opportunity to clarify and cope with issues so that they do not consume her thoughts once the baby arrives. And it can lead to a healthy acceptance of the physical changes. A pregnant woman may not be ecstatic about her bulging belly, swollen feet and gastrointestinal discomfort. But she can at least accept that the changes of pregnancy are only temporary and that millions of other expectant mothers are also experiencing them.

Finally, if a woman is no longer agonizing over her "inability" to become that stereotypical beaming pregnant woman, she is free to concentrate on some of the more important tasks at hand: becoming a mother, and taking care of herself and her child.

MYTH #2: Having a baby can save a strained marriage

Many couples are under the misimpression that having a baby can fix or even save a troubled marriage. Yet, the role renegotiations required to respond to the unremitting demands of a new infant, coupled with the loss of time, energy and freedom, can strain even the strongest of relationships, as new couples find themselves trying to create order amidst chaos. A number of studies have documented a sharp decline in marital satisfaction following the birth of a first child.[5-7] Jealousy and resentment may arise, loyalties can shift, and a new parent may feel as if the baby is intruding upon the well-established rhythms of the marital relationship. Factor in a lack of sleep and insecurities about one's ability to care competently for an infant, and new parents are primed for a fight. They are ready to lash out at the first person they see: most likely, each other.

Jim and Janine went through an unanticipated rough patch after their son, Nathan, was born. Janine says people warned her that marital dynamics change once the baby arrives, but she did not believe them. She recalls her reaction to their comments: "'Oh well, it's not going to happen to me and Jim. We get along so well, and he's going to be a great dad. We talk about things. That's not going to happen to us.' And sure enough, it did … I never expected to bicker and fight over the stupid things that we do because we never did that before. I thought, 'Oh, we have such a good foundation. It's going to be great.' I can't imagine what happens to a couple who doesn't have a good foundation like we do and can't necessarily talk these things out. I can't imagine the kind of stress this would bring to their relationship."

MYTH #3: Children are destined to repeat their parents' mistakes

Having a child is a chance to start anew. It is an opportunity for a parent to reflect on his (or her) own upbringing, to understand his earliest childhood experiences. This reflection may help him identify what his parents failed to provide on an emotional level and clarify what he would like to do differently with his own children. An awareness of these experiences and their significance can empower an expectant or new parent by helping him realize that he can make different parenting choices than the ones his parents made. This type of introspection can also help heal old wounds.

Over and over again, the expectant and new parents interviewed for this book talked about how their own parents were physically and/or emotionally absent from their lives. Having experienced this, they understood what they wanted to offer their own children: love, support and attention, all intangible but invaluable. In fact, a number of the fathers interviewed said they had changed jobs or scaled back their work schedules in order to spend more time with their children.

MYTH #4: Life will not be that different once the baby arrives

Many expectant parents assume that after the baby is born, life will be the same as it was before, except with a child in the house. They do not anticipate the enormity of the changes they are about to experience as they move from being a couple to a family. They fail to contemplate how the increased demands on their time and the loss of freedom will affect their relationships and their every-day lives. Even eating a meal together as a couple requires major planning.

A new baby can be all-consuming, but many expectant mothers and fathers believe their infants will do nothing but sleep and eat during those first few weeks, leaving them (the parents) essentially to go about their lives as before. Although most people understand that they will have additional responsibilities as parents, they are not necessarily aware of just how much extra work one little person creates. There is always one more bottle to be sterilized, yet another load of stained baby clothes to be washed, or a last-minute diaper run to be made.

Parents-to-be cannot possibly predict every change that will occur once the baby is born, but they can be fairly certain their lives will be markedly different. Some things they will not or cannot know, such as whether they will really want to return to work full-time. A new parent may decide to stay at home, cut back her hours or shift to a more flexible work schedule. Also expectant parents do not necessarily know ahead of time how involved their parents and in-laws will be in their lives once the baby arrives. After all, most people cannot seem to stay away from a new baby. And new parents might find all of that togetherness intrusive, as relatives descend upon their home, dispensing advice on the "right way" to take care of an infant.

Many expectant parents vow that their newborns will never share a room with them. It is a nice idea in theory but one that is not always practical in the real world of new parenthood. Once the baby is born, and parents spend several nights traipsing over to his room every few hours to feed him, they may recognize that an all-in-one-room sleeping arrangement makes overnight baby care a more low-maintenance affair. After all, it requires far less energy to reach for a crying baby parked in a bassinet next to one's bed than it does to trek down a hallway to the nursery. (Real estate is not the only area in which the mantra "location, location, location" applies.) But one of the drawbacks of the "family bedroom" is that it can encroach upon a couple's privacy – probably not an issue they had to worry about when it was just the two of them.

MYTH #5: The maternal instinct

The "maternal instinct," a term embedded in the language of our culture, suggests that new mothers always know exactly what their babies need. For example, it assumes that a new mother can determine, from the moment of birth, precisely what each cry means and how she should respond. The myth of the maternal instinct implies that every aspect of mothering is like some involuntary reflex, that it is natural and automatic for all women. But like any other relationship, it often takes time for an emotional connection to develop between a mother and her infant. When a woman first meets her future husband, she does not know everything about him (and vice versa). She has not had time to learn his pet peeves or preferences. She does not know how he likes his steak cooked, or whether he is the type of man who cries every time he watches one of the quintessential male tearjerker films such as *Field of Dreams* or *Brian's Song*. And she is incapable of interpreting the nuances of his behavior. That all takes time, and it is no different with a baby. Those who fault themselves for not immediately knowing how to soothe their babies or decode their distress signals can end up feeling as if they have somehow failed their children. But parenting is a work in progress.

In addition, men, who are generally not conditioned to see themselves as nurturers and caregivers, may also buy into the myth of the maternal instinct. These men see their wives as having a sort of "baby omniscience." So when their babies cry, they tend to sit back and let their wives, "the experts," soothe them.

MYTH #6: Maternal bonding

The myth of the maternal instinct implies that a mother always knows what her baby needs and how she should respond. The myth of maternal bonding suggests that a new mother will have an instant, electro-charged connection with her baby, and that as soon as the baby comes out of her womb, she will fall in love with him. A mother and her baby have an emerging, evolving relationship. They do not necessarily establish the rhythms of this relationship overnight. The "instant" part of maternal bonding has been greatly exaggerated. Although some women do feel an immediate and overwhelming emotional connection to their babies, others do not.

Shannon, a Boston mother of twin boys, spent five years trying to have children, experiencing the emotional roller-coaster ride so common in the world of fertility treatments. Yet even after all her efforts and all of her heartache, she did not bond with her boys right away. "You have to fall in love with them, though I guess what was surprising was that it wasn't instantaneous for me. It was instantaneous the feeling that I needed to care for them, but it's just been a process of falling in love with them. And I think every day I just love them a little more."

Maggie, a new mom from New Jersey, expresses a similar sentiment. She talks about her friends' experiences: "From the moment they saw their children, they just had this amazing feeling of love," says Maggie. "They never thought they could love anything as much ... I just didn't have that same overwhelming feeling just from that immediate moment. I had read enough to know that a lot of people don't feel that way. But if I hadn't read about that, I think I would've thought something was wrong with me."

LeeRan was born in Korea and adopted by a Caucasian family from Minnesota when she was 6 months old. She could not wait to have a baby so that she might have a family member who actually looked like her. Yet she says that when her son Matthew was born, "I didn't have that aching for or that bond with this baby until I would say about three weeks postpartum."

MYTH #7: The average baby

Every baby is as unique as her fingerprints. No two babies have the exact same temperament, sleep patterns or eating habits. Nor do they develop at the same pace. It is natural for a nervous new parent to compare his baby with others, in order to confirm that his baby is "on track" and to make sure that, as a parent, he is doing what he is supposed to do. But new mothers and fathers get too caught up in comparisons and averages. Parameters outlined in parenting books and by organizations such as the American Academy of Pediatrics are written to help parents determine when they might want to consult their own pediatricians; they do not necessarily indicate that something is wrong if a baby's behavior falls outside those guidelines.

"That's why guidelines are just that, guidelines," notes Dr. Palmo Pasquariello, a pediatrician in Manhattan. He says, for example, there are some babies who will not sleep the expected 18 to 20 hours a day in the first few weeks. "Sleep *guidelines* were always something of a little joke to me because guidelines are what work for you," he remarks. However, he says that if parents notice that their baby's sleep pattern does appear extremely disrupted, they should speak with the child's doctor.

A new parent who reads too much into averages may be needlessly disappointed. Even seemingly innocuous comments from others, such as "Most babies sleep through the night at six months," or "Most babies have a special security blanket or toy for comfort," can make a parent feel inadequate if his child is not one of those babies. But, as Dr. Pasquariello so aptly declares, "There is no such thing as a textbook child. The textbook child lives only in a textbook."

MYTH #8: The perfect parent

Who is the perfect parent? He or she exists only as a figment of our imagination. Yet so many of us strive to become this fictitious character who provides all that a child requires and desires, and who can virtually guarantee her child's happiness and success. She is always willing to make whatever sacrifices necessary to support her children. The perfect parent is so in tune with her children that she can even anticipate what they need and want. She knows how to help her kids through every conceivable situation. She is a skilled disciplinarian who recognizes when to tighten the reins and when to loosen them.

In addition, the perfect parent quickly masters whatever parenting methods the experts are currently espousing. But as she diligently attempts to follow their advice to a tee, she may be doing herself and her child a disservice. In effect, she has transferred her authority as the best expert on her own child to these various childcare gurus, instead of trusting her own instincts and common sense. This is not to say that some of the experts' parenting books cannot be helpful. (We hope this one is.) But every child is different, every parent is different, and what is best for one child and parent might not be appropriate for another.

Lastly, there is something wrong with even thinking it is possible for a new parent to attain perfection. How can one be skilled, let alone perfect, at something one has never done before? Think about that first job after college. Most of us made mistakes, and then had a colleague discreetly take us aside to show us the ropes before anyone else discovered we were not yet on top of things. Yet, the fear of making mistakes paralyzes some new mothers and fathers and interferes with the process of building self-confidence in the capacity to parent. Parenting is about trial and error. And it is sometimes the errors that teach us how to be better parents, albeit not perfect ones.

CHAPTER 2

The mind–body connection of pregnancy

Mother Nature has a way of forcing expectant couples to acknowledge the profound roles they are about to assume. A swelling belly, puffy feet, morning sickness, exhaustion, and those first few fetal kicks are all part of the physiological experience of pregnancy that inevitably gives rise to the expectant couple's psychological experience. The two are inextricably linked. The transformations taking place in the woman's body are often the couple's first tangible connection to parenthood, the first emotional tie to the growing baby within. These powerful physical changes can influence the way a woman views her body. They can also affect how an expectant couple feels about intimacy and impending parenthood. Both women and men may discover that some of the physical aspects of pregnancy have them oscillating between contradictory emotions, for pregnancy can be both joyous and stressful, both frightening and awe-inspiring. For example, a couple may be ecstatic after seeing the first ultrasound, but then apprehensive, wondering how they will measure up as parents. A woman may be excited about becoming a mother, but upset by her expanding waistline. Most new parents will get a healthy taste of this emotional cocktail.

The psychological journey to parenthood has no precise timeline and does not follow a set path. So, even though some expectant parents start to feel connected to their unborn babies extremely early in the pregnancy – at the first doctor's appointment or with the mother's inaugural bout of nausea – others do not establish that tie until much later. Regardless of when it occurs, this initial emotional link signals that the baby is more than just a theoretical being represented by a red line on a pregnancy test. Rather, it is a real person for whom they will be responsible and who will eventually call them "mom" and "dad." So, in a sense, physical gestation is also a time of psychological gestation for expectant mothers and fathers as they make the transition to parenthood.

For Stacey, the reality of impending motherhood set in when her pants became too tight. Her stomach had just started to bulge, and she was feeling the first few flutters of tiny feet. She then began to feel "protective" of her stomach and connected to the baby inside. For Nakisha, the ultrasound scan, tiny movements from within, and a new fullness to her normally tiny figure made the baby more real for her. She notes, "I looked the same, but bloated, so it was like, 'Something's really in there, you know?'" Marla, from California, says that when her husband, Bryan, first heard their son's heartbeat, he cried "like a baby." "It was very moving," says Bryan. "I always pictured myself as a father, I always wondered what it would be like to be a father, and then it was happening. I really didn't know what to feel. It was kind of surreal." Similarly, 35-year-old Ralph says, "For a first-time dad, you get that surreal feeling. But also you don't really know what's going on until you go to that first sonogram appointment and you see your little baby in there. Up until that point, from a father's perspective, there's nothing really too different other than that you take care of your wife a little bit more." Ralph's wife, Vanessa, describes him as a big fan of sonograms. "He always wanted to get one. He'd say, 'Are we getting a sonogram at today's appointment?' It made him feel closer to the baby to actually see her." Especially for fathers-to-be, a sonogram is the kind of picture that is definitely worth more than a thousand words. Jan Draper, a Programme Director with the Royal College of Nursing Institute, conducted a study on men's experiences of becoming fathers. She found that the ultrasound scan brought men "right into the centre of the action" by heightening their awareness of their babies. She concluded that, for a man, the ultrasound images "reinforced" the reality that his transition to fatherhood had begun.[8]

Leslie,* a physician, says a dream she had two weeks before the 20-week ultrasound helped her form an emotional connection to her unborn baby. "As silly as it sounds, I had a dream one night about a little boy who looked exactly like my husband," remarks Leslie. "And – lo and behold – two weeks later we found out it was a boy. I had just gotten it in my head that it was a boy after I had that dream. So every time he kicked or punched, I imagined him playing soccer or fighting with another little boy or something like that. I imagined him being aggressive and assertive – not that a little girl wouldn't be, because my parents tell me I was a hellion!"

Paul literally needed a good kick in the head before he could fully appreciate the idea that he and Kate were going to become parents. Resting his head on Kate's pregnant stomach one day, little Elliot punted him. "That was reality," declares Paul. "The baby was moving and *I* felt it. And it really brought it home for me." Prior to the head-kicking episode, "It was just Katy saying, 'Oh, I can feel it, I can feel it.'"

A father gets to know his unborn child

In Paul's opinion, biology has afforded women the home-court advantage when it comes to connecting with their unborn children. Women are privy to their babies' every kick, flip and hiccup. Consequently, they begin to get to know

---

*Some names have been changed at the request of interviewees.

their babies – what makes them squirm around, what gives them gas, and what pacifies them. "I think there's a risk of, not the man feeling left out, but not being able to connect with the baby, whereas I think Katy connected with Elliot before he was born," comments Paul.

Men can bond with their unborn children in a number of ways. They can talk or sing to them. They can read stories to them. Dr. Thomas Verny is one of the pioneers in the field of perinatal psychology. He emphasizes that an unborn baby, especially after the sixth month, has an "active emotional life" inside the womb, that he can feel emotions, as well as hear, touch, taste and smell.

Verny says, "Once parents really, really comprehend ... that this baby is more than just a blob of protoplasm, that from the beginning it has tremendous potential, ... [that] certainly from the end of the second trimester, it is a sensing, feeling, aware and remembering human being ... then I think everything else really follows from it because then you do treat the baby with the respect that a human being deserves, instead of as just a blob of protoplasm, like some kind of a goldfish in a bowl of water." He adds, "We know that children are able to differentiate their mothers' voices from other mothers' voices as soon as they are born, and that they are able to appreciate also their fathers' voices if their fathers have spoken to them."

Neonatologist Frederick Wirth teaches parents how to communicate with their unborn babies in his book, *Prenatal Parenting: The Complete Psychological and Spiritual Guide to Loving Your Unborn Child.*[9] He says that by using a simple test, he can determine whether a father has "been active" in communicating with his unborn child. Dr. Wirth writes, "I do this by holding the infant between me and his father while we compete for the infant's attention by calling the child's name. If the dad has been actively involved in the reading and singing, his child will turn his head toward him, looking for the source of the sound. Invariably, when their eyes meet they both react positively."[9]

Bryan, a father from Laguna Beach, California, was proud of his ability to communicate with his unborn baby and pleased that he alone could calm his son. He observed, "It's so weird, but when Marla puts her hand where he's kicking, he kicks more. When I do it, he gets quiet immediately." This kind of special interaction between an expectant father and his unborn child is an important element of his emerging identity as a father.

Body image

During pregnancy, there are the women who glow, the women who glower, and the men who love them. Some women truly enjoy being pregnant. Pregnancy is the ultimate embodiment of their womanhood. A woman who "glows" may see every pound she gains as just another reminder of the wonderful life she is carrying. The additional weight sometimes brings a newfound sensuality as she becomes more voluptuous. She may also experience a greater sense of freedom; for once, she is able to give herself permission to take a break from the pressures of dieting, stringent workouts and always having to fit into her "skinny" jeans.

But not all expectant mothers find the pregnancy experience enjoyable. Expectant mothers may feel big, uncomfortable, ugly and even angry. One study of pregnant women found that weight gain, body changes and physical distresses, including nausea, vomiting and fatigue, were among the most common stressors.[10] Nothing upsets some women more than watching the numbers on the scale jump higher and higher into uncharted territory. For a woman who finds the physical transformations of pregnancy difficult or unpleasant, seeing her own reflection in the mirror can be a daunting experience, particularly if she has not been able to let go of her pre-pregnancy preoccupation with appearance. She may feel a loss of control because she cannot manage her body the way she could before her pregnancy. And she may be left wondering, "Am I still attractive? Will I ever get my body back?"

Men are also divided when it comes to their opinions about the physical changes of pregnancy. They may be asking themselves different questions, such as "When will my wife look, feel and act like she did before the pregnancy?" Some men do not find the transformation appealing. Others are in awe at the sight of their partners' blossoming bodies carrying their precious babies. Furthermore, an expectant father may see the growing baby as the ultimate embodiment of the love he shares with his partner.

A lot has happened in the past few decades to influence the ways both men and women view the pregnant body. Women's increased presence in the workforce, their growing confidence at having secured places there, and the showcasing of celebrity pregnancies have all altered our perceptions. In our culture today, the pregnant form is something that can be displayed proudly, rather than covered up by a voluminous tent dress, or in the case of Princess Grace Kelly back in 1956, a strategically placed Hermès bag. Kelly, who was photographed with the bag positioned to conceal her pregnant stomach, created such a sensation with her creative "maternity wear" that the French luxury goods maker quickly named the bag after her. Designer handbags aside, by the early 1980s, women needed a suitable clothing option that was appropriate for their roles as expectant mothers and professionals, in a work environment where the welcome mat was not always readily set out.

In 1982, Rebecca Matthias was pregnant with her first child and could not find decent maternity clothes to wear to work. So she did something about it. She started her own catalog business to try to fill that market void. Her first catalog featured maternity clothes for professional women, including a navy blue suit she created. "My best product was my little navy blue suit," notes Matthias. Catering to the "conceal-your-pregnancy" mentality, she designed the suit to hide the obvious signs of pregnancy. "When you were a high-powered professional woman and you got pregnant, you didn't want the boss to know about it because he wouldn't take you seriously," she says. "So we all dressed in navy blue suits with little red bow-ties. We wanted to look like men. And that's what put me in business. This was a whole new wave. Before, women hadn't worked through their pregnancies." Out of her own experience as a mother-to-be, Matthias, along with her husband, took that little navy blue suit, and the catalog in which it was featured, and developed her company into the world's largest maternity retailer, *Mothers Work, Inc.*, parent company to *A Pea in the Pod, Mimi Maternity, Motherhood Maternity* and *Destination Maternity*.

"Clothes to me are a reflection of society and what's going on in society," she notes. Since the formation of her company more than a quarter of a century ago, Matthias has been perched in a unique position to observe how women view their pregnant bodies. She says they have gone from hiding them, to flaunting them, a trend that has paralleled the growing numbers of women in the labor force. She explains, "As women became more confident, and it was taken for granted that they worked in the office and everywhere else, then we came back to being sexy. ... So I think when they felt more entitled, then they felt more confident and they felt like they could dress in a more feminine way."

An even more recent factor has strongly influenced the way people perceive the pregnant body: the pregnant celebrity. She is hard to miss. In the past decade, the rich and famous have started to display their pregnant figures for all the world to admire and photograph. It has become difficult to pass a newsstand without catching a glimpse of some pregnant star – Cindy Crawford, various Spice Girls, Elizabeth Hurley and, more recently, Britney Spears. They have helped make pregnancy panache a reality instead of a contradiction, and they have glamorized the road to motherhood. These pregnant celebrities have shown us that the pregnant body is something to celebrate and that a woman need not give up her sense of style just because she is now dressing for two. No tent dresses for these women!

But there is also a downside to celebrities' exhibitions of motherhood-in-the-making. As is often the case when we take our cues from these well-known names, we end up creating unrealistic expectations for the general population in this instance, the general population of pregnant women. Many expectant celebrities, always ready to strike a pose for the paparazzi, are only too proud to show off their svelte silhouettes (save for slightly bulging mid-sections). This can leave the pregnant woman who does gain more than 20 pounds feeling self-conscious about her changing physique. The phenomenon of the famous bearing their pregnant bellies has idealized pregnancy and given credence to the myth that pregnancy is the happiest time for all women, a time when they never looked or felt better. What many people do not realize is that practically any woman can glow if she has an unlimited budget to spend on designer maternity wear, as well as a professional hair stylist and make-up artist. Because of this emphasis on achieving a sort of "Barbie-doll pregnancy," women tend to forget that weight gain is a normal part of a healthy pregnancy. The American College of Obstetricians and Gynecologists recommends that women gain 25 to 35 pounds during pregnancy, a little more if they start out underweight, or a little less if they are overweight.[11]

It is the combination of these factors – women's established place in the workforce, the glamorization of pregnancy and the creation of unrealistic ideals for the female form – that affects how men and women view the pregnant body today. Forty-year-old Catherine was one of the glowers. "I loved the clothes I wore. I always felt attractive. I always felt like a good-looking pregnant woman. I still felt sexy. I actually felt more so in some ways. I felt more womanly, and I felt very good about it. And I enjoyed the attention I got for looking good," says the Los Angeles mother. Her husband, Mark, exclaims, "To see her grow was fantastic, and I really hadn't known how I was going to feel about it. I had no idea."

Catherine says even though she enjoyed her pregnant body, she worried, "'Am I going to gain 80 pounds and throw up like crazy? Am I not going to be able to stop gaining weight?' ... But I didn't have any problems like those, and I didn't try to avoid gaining weight or have the attitude, 'Well, I'll just have a scoop of tuna and some carrots.' No, no. I ate well. But if I wanted a cheeseburger and fries, I got a cheeseburger and fries." Twenty-seven-year-old Ginette also says pregnancy made her feel attractive. "I'm on the heavy side, and I've never had a great love of my body. But there I was, pregnant, and I didn't care. It was me and my daughter, and it was great!" she declares.

Like Catherine and Ginette, Stacey did not mind gaining weight during her pregnancy. "I was happy when the doctor said, 'Oh, you've gained five pounds. You've gained eight pounds.' That to me was great. I knew the pregnancy was going well. I was gaining the weight for the baby, and I figured that at some point I'd lose it. I just hoped that it wouldn't take me too long." She continues, laughing, "I liked the fact that my boobs were bigger. That was one bonus. I kind of miss that a little." Having her husband's support was a big confidence booster. "He never said things such as, 'Oh my God, your butt's so big.' He loved watching me grow and feeling my stomach. So that helped, that he wasn't turned off by my shape," comments Stacey. Her husband, Loren, states, "I thought it made her more beautiful than she was before. Absolutely I noticed the changes, but I didn't think of her as any less beautiful physically."

Jodi, a massage therapist, did not exactly embrace her pregnant body, but admits acquiescing to a healthy acceptance of what was happening. "I had to surrender to the fact that my body was going to change, and I had to stop trying to fight it," she says. Meanwhile, Jodi's husband, David, confesses that he has always found pregnant women attractive. "I think it's very sexy, you know, the glow. It seems like a woman is more complete when she's pregnant." Jodi, eight months pregnant, proudly recounts the story of a male bonding trip that any pregnant woman would be delighted to hear: "David was in Vegas last weekend with his friends, and the guys took him to a strip club – that doesn't bother me at all, and it grosses him out. Later he said, 'You know, I kept thinking about how beautiful my wife is. I'd rather be watching my wife right now.'"

Pregnancy weight gain is a considerable source of stress for many women, especially those who were particularly focused on staying trim prior to pregnancy. Keri, mother of 5-month-old Cooper, found it difficult to see her carefully maintained figure take on an additional 52 pounds during pregnancy. "I have always been a fit person. I exercised throughout the whole pregnancy. It was hard for me to see myself gain so much weight. I felt really insecure. I didn't want D.J. to ever see me without my clothes on," says the Kentucky mother. Keri states that whenever she had to change her clothes or get ready to take a shower, she would hide from her husband. "Now I look back," she reflects, "and wish I had embraced the pregnancy a little bit more. And the next time we have a child, I will embrace it more and not worry so much about how much weight I'm gaining or how I look."

Meanwhile, D.J. notes that although he was never "one of those guys" who thinks that "all pregnant women are beautiful," he was pleasantly surprised when he saw Keri's pregnant body. "Once I saw my wife pregnant with my baby, it was amazingly beautiful. I got caught up in the whole romantic idea of her carrying our baby and God putting a miracle inside her and watching her grow, which meant watching him grow. It was so exciting."

When 22-year-old Emily from Cheshire, England, was first interviewed, she was six months pregnant and very upset about the changes she had been seeing in her body. "I've put on a lot of weight, one and a half stone [21 pounds]. I've got stretch marks. ... I definitely don't like the way my body is developing. Having a bigger bust and the stretch marks, I don't feel as confident," she says. Emily believes that her feelings about her body have colored her outlook on becoming a mother. "When I feel very low or down about myself, I think more about what I would be like if I wasn't pregnant, that I'd be this outgoing, bubbly person."

Valerie, a mother from Cleveland, also struggled with the weight gain. "I have always been around a size 6, size 8. I never really had to watch what I ate and never really gained weight. ... I had a decent body image and then all of a sudden, I was getting fat. And I really, really, really had a hard time with that." Unlike Stacey, Valerie was not a fan of her tight pants. "I remember the first week in March. I put my jeans on, and then two days later I had an inch gap. And that was really hard for me because I felt like I was getting fat."

Valerie's husband, Brett, says he would include himself in the "pregnancy-is-beautiful" category, but diplomatically qualifies: "It's quite a change in the female body. I'd say anything up to five months is a very cute look. But then as the baby grows inside and [the woman] gets larger, especially when she gets to the end of the third trimester, it's like, 'Let's hurry up and get the baby born so you can get your body back to normal.' ... As a guy, I'm thinking, 'I'm glad I don't have to go through that.'"

Kate has always viewed other pregnant women as "absolutely stunning."

"But I didn't feel that for myself," she notes, clarifying, "I just didn't think that I looked nice ... I didn't want to spend the money on nice clothes for myself. If I had spent some money on nice clothes, then maybe I might have felt better." Kate says she probably went overboard wearing big, loose-fitting clothes to cover up her pregnant shape. "My neighbors didn't realize I was pregnant. And then I came home with this baby and they were like, 'Where did that come from?'" she recalls. "I wish I had just worn some more fitted clothes and shown people my tummy."

Beyond the weight gain

Weight gain is the most obvious physical change of pregnancy. But other changes, including stretch marks, morning sickness, fatigue, as well as hundreds of pregnancy-related medical conditions, can also influence how expectant parents feel about the pregnancy, and how they connect to their baby before he is born. These changes also play a role in the amount of stress expectant parents experience during those nine months.

Wande, mother of 10-month-old England, suffered terrible morning sickness. "It was constant. It wasn't like once a day. It was like five or six times a day," she explains. The nausea and vomiting lasted until about three weeks before England was born. The Atlanta mom says jokingly, "I thought God was getting me back for the way I treated my mom. I swear. I said, 'God is getting me back for the awful things I did to my mom.' I was Satan's child."

When she was eight months pregnant, Wande went into premature labor, so her doctor put her on bed rest. That did not sit well with her. "I'm a get-up-and-go person," she says. "I need to be on the move. I get cabin fever after a few hours in the house. So for me, when I was physically not able to do anything and forced to stay in the house, forced to stay in bed all day, it just wasn't fun." Being a "get-up-and-go" person, Wande got up and went, despite her doctor's orders. She explains, "I listened to him for about a day, and then I was climbing the stairs, driving around, going to church. I couldn't deny England church. She really kicked when I took her [there]. I think she liked the music."

Thirty-two weeks into her pregnancy, Kate began to feel itchy on her hands, feet and arms, and then all over her body. She was diagnosed with obstetric cholestasis, which causes an accumulation of bile acids in the bloodstream. According to Dr. Gila Leiter, an obstetrician and gynecologist in New York City, cholestasis can be "a marker for complications of pregnancy. And so we make sure that the babies are growing properly, that there's no increase in preterm labor, growth-restricted fetuses, et cetera," notes Dr. Leiter, adding that the condition is associated with a "slight increased risk of stillbirth."

Kate says discovering that she had a condition that could potentially threaten the life of her unborn baby was "horrific." "I just tried to be brave for Paul [her husband], and he tried to be brave for me, neither of us knowing what was going on." Kate and Paul understood that there was a good chance doctors would induce her before the due date because of the risks associated with obstetric cholestasis. Paul describes, "It was a very long process because the doctors and nurses told us that from that day onward, she could be put in the hospital. At any time, she could've been called in. So the overnight bag went into the car and we were ready to go, and we were on tenterhooks waiting day in and day out."

Jennifer says that in addition to unsightly stretch marks which made her "cry and cry and cry," she came down with a horrible case of PUPPP (pruritic urticarial papules and plaques of pregnancy) rash that typically occurs during the last trimester, but which she developed in her third month. It continued for the remainder of her pregnancy. "It was basically like having poison ivy all over my body. It was everywhere but my face and the soles of my feet and the palms of my hands," says Jennifer. "Sometimes I would end up taking several oatmeal baths a night [to relieve the itchiness]." Asked if she felt resentful because of the rash, the stretch marks and the discomfort of carrying twins, Jennifer answered, "You know who I was mad at was Fred. I just felt like he had no idea how miserable I was, and then I was angry because he didn't have to do anything. It was like, 'Well, I'm glad you're so happy about these children. I'm the one who's suffering to give them to you.'" She added, "But I have to say he was an angel putting cream on me every time I woke up. He also helped me out of the bath because I couldn't get out by myself." Of Jennifer's difficult pregnancy, Fred says, "It was hard, not just from a sympathy standpoint. She was kind of a pain to be around. It made her attitude difficult. I was even worried about when the babies came. I tried to tell her, 'Oh, it's all going to be worth it when the babies come.' But she didn't really want to hear that at the time."

Unfortunately, husbands and partners tend to bear the brunt of pregnant women's frustrations. Women are inclined to consider their significant others "safe" outlets for their anger. After all, men are not the ones "suffering," as Jennifer put it, to create a family. But some men do experience physical symptoms of pregnancy. They just do it without being pregnant.

Couvade syndrome

The term "couvade" is derived from the French word *couver*, meaning "to hatch." Though not well understood, couvade syndrome is known as "sympathetic pregnancy." Men with couvade syndrome experience physical symptoms of pregnancy – including various gastrointestinal disturbances, weight gain, and aches and pains – that have no physiological basis.[12] Studies indicate that more than 50% of men may experience some symptoms of couvade syndrome.[13]

Bryan explains how Marla's pregnancy made him feel: "Whenever she would wake up, I would wake up. Whenever she would hurt, I would hurt. We were just kind of on the same wavelength for a long time." Bryan ended up putting on 30 pounds, which falls within the American College of Obstetricians and Gynecologists' recommended weight gain for pregnant *women*!

Sex during pregnancy

Sexual intimacy during pregnancy is an extremely sensitive subject for some couples, making for particularly awkward discussions. It is as if an unease that previously never existed infiltrates the most private arena of a couple's life together. While some couples boast that pregnancy greatly enhances their sexual experiences, others shy away from intercourse, for fear of hurting the baby, causing the woman discomfort or initiating early labor. In addition, the baby, although tucked away in the uterus, may be seen as intruding on the couple's privacy.

A woman's desire to have sex can change throughout her pregnancy. During the first trimester, nausea, vomiting, fatigue and fluctuating hormone levels can contribute to a decreased sex drive. In the second trimester, women typically experience a welcome burst of energy, and the nausea and vomiting tend to decrease, if not disappear altogether. Obstetrician Gila Leiter, who has been delivering babies for 23 years, says, "As the second trimester begins, this tends to be the best time for interest in intercourse and increased sexuality. Many women are happy with their body image in the second trimester; their breasts are a little bit larger, they feel good, they certainly feel better than in the first trimester." But once a couple enters the third trimester, interest in sexual intercourse may wane again. This is when the aches and pains of pregnancy tend to be especially prominent. A woman may no longer be comfortable, physically or emotionally, with her larger body. Consequently, she may be embarrassed about being sexually intimate with her own husband. One study found that women's desire to have sex diminishes during the course of pregnancy, especially in the last three months. The study also showed a marked increase in the number of men who experienced a diminished sex drive in the third trimester.[14] Yet Dr. Leiter says some women "continue to have a great interest in sex right until delivery is more imminent."

Neil likes to joke that his sex life is non-existent, but his pregnant wife, Robin, declares, "We definitely are still having sex, but just less frequently!" Entering her second trimester, Robin says nausea and fatigue curbed her enthusiasm during the first three months. "I have a long day at work. And so all I really have the energy for is to eat dinner and go to sleep. It's hard enough to just get through the work day ... I'm more in the mood to have sex on the weekends. I have more energy because I didn't work all day. I think that's a big part of it."

Neil says, "There have certainly been times when I may have wanted to have sex, but she just wasn't feeling up to it." He explains how he copes: "I think my mentality has changed a little bit. I just don't even really think it's something that's going to happen. So I just sort of put it out of my mind, and then occasionally we try to make it work. And we've been able to do that, but it's definitely a different flow." He adds, "The one thing that I think I have to be a little bit careful of is to make sure I'm not pressing on her stomach, because that can cause a little discomfort for her."

Kelly and Roberto were able to maintain a scaled-down version of their sex life even though it became uncomfortable for her. Three-and-a-half months before giving birth, Kelly notes, "What sucks is that sex hurts. I haven't really been able to have any good sex because everything is so engorged inside. So I'm jealous of these women who say (squealing), 'Oh, it's so great. Oh my God.'" She continues, "But I feel sexy! I don't know what it is. Men just come up to me, and they want to touch my belly. I'm getting so much attention that I love it!"

One of her biggest admirers is her husband. Roberto boasts, "She's a sexy, hot mama ... I love it, I love it! I don't know what it is because some part of [pregnancy] is so sacred. But at the same time it's so raw, it's so sexy, it's so sexual. I freak out because I think, 'Oh my God, am I a pervert or something?' ... And her breasts." "I was already big," chimes in Kelly. "But I've grown half a size around, and I've grown one-and-a-half or two cup sizes."

When Wande went into labor early, her doctor advised her to stop having intercourse. Up until then, Wande and Dino had had a very active sex life. "When I was seven months pregnant, we were like jack-rabbits," she remarks. Dr. Leiter says sexual activity during a low-risk pregnancy is fine, but when a woman has a condition such as placenta previa, or other complications, including vaginal bleeding and preterm labor, it is best for her to refrain from having intercourse.

Nakisha was two months pregnant when she got the news that she had placenta previa, a condition in which the placenta covers the cervix. "It could have caused me to hemorrhage," she explains, "so I wasn't allowed to have sex."

D.J. worried that having sexual intercourse with Keri would initiate labor early. "On these TV shows, they always talk about sex as a way of expediting delivery and getting labor kick-started. And I was probably thinking, 'God, she's only 28 weeks. What if this causes her to go into labor early?'" Also, for D.J., three was a crowd. Knowing that baby Cooper was right there in the room with them, albeit inside his wife's womb with an obstructed view, made him uneasy. D.J. says, "I'm the first to admit, it was all me, and I was completely weirded out, even after her doctors' urgings. They would say, 'Don't worry about it. ... You're not going to hurt anybody, you can't do any damage where the baby is.' ... But him being up there, the whole thing didn't seem like fun to me."

Like Keri's doctors who tried to set D.J.'s mind at ease, Dr. Leiter says that unless there are complications with the pregnancy, sex does not hurt the baby or the woman. But a pregnant woman should "appreciate and respect her comfort zone," she advises. "If it feels uncomfortable, the position isn't comfortable or if she feels a lot of pressure, then she has to be more creative, use extra lubrication or change positions. Lots of women use different positions during pregnancy," positions they did not regularly use before pregnancy.

So can sexual intercourse initiate labor? Dr. Leiter says not unless the cervix is already dilated: "In a low-risk pregnancy with a long, closed cervix, there is no increase in premature labor related to sexual intercourse." In a study published in 2001, researchers at the University of North Carolina at Chapel Hill found that sexual activity between 29 and 36 weeks did not cause premature delivery.[15]

Fears of causing premature labor, of hurting the baby and/or woman, and of the baby being "aware" that the couple is having sexual intercourse are just a few of the reasons a man might feel awkward about his physical relationship with the mother of his unborn child. But David had a different concern. "It was funny," he recalls, "I was very hands-off with Jodi. I was hands-off and it bummed her out ... I just sort of got like, 'Wow, she's carrying our child' ... I guess it was what they call the Madonna [Whore] complex." Some of the more recent psychological literature discusses the Madonna–Whore complex in terms of a man's internal conflict in continuing to view his partner as a sexual being as she moves through pregnancy to motherhood. In this context, a mother is pure and virginal, not a sexual figure to be lusted after.[16] Grappling with this paradox requires an awareness of the profound mind-body connection of pregnancy.

That same awareness can open the door to a better understanding of the transition to parenthood. A mother's protruding stomach, the sonogram, and even nausea and modified sexual activity can all lead to a heightened focus on the unborn baby who is about to make her way into the world. This awareness may ignite a yearning to forge an emotional connection with her. An expectant couple may start to think about what kind of personality their baby will have. They may begin to wonder what she will look like, whether she will have her father's nose or her mother's eyes. And they may amuse themselves by trying to guess where her talents may lie and what she will be when she grows up. But pregnancy is not only the perfect time to think about the baby, it is also the ideal time to think about being a parent.

CHAPTER 3

Motherhood: the psychological experience

Most women would not dream of going through nine months of pregnancy without the requisite prenatal care – regular doctors' appointments, special vitamins, a well-balanced diet, and diagnostic tests to check on the health of the baby. Yet they do not devote nearly the same amount of time or attention, if any, to the psychological aspects of impending motherhood. They fail to recognize how this profound role they are about to assume will alter their lives forever.

Typically, when a woman plans for life after pregnancy, she considers only her work and childcare arrangements. By the last trimester, she has probably already lined up a nanny or selected a day-care center, or at least thought about it. She also may have arranged for a more flexible work schedule in order to meet the demands of her new family life, which is just around the corner. But women generally do not take the time to reflect on the journey to motherhood, although they seem to have plenty of time to attend prenatal Pilates classes and register for the latest baby paraphernalia. They do not stop to ask them-selves, "Am I ready to become a mother? What are my biggest fears regarding motherhood? What might it be like to stay at home alone with a newborn all day during those first few months? How can I begin to integrate and prioritize my different roles? And what does my relationship with my own mother have to do with any of this?"

Today much has been made of the "supermom" phenomenon, the pressure for a woman to achieve perfection in each of her roles – mother, wife and professional. As a result, many women approach motherhood in overdrive, believing they must "accomplish" something at every point along the path to parenthood. The ideal pregnancy is one in which a woman exercises such control over her body that she does not need to wear maternity clothes until her eighth month. The gold standard for labor and delivery is a quick, easy, epidural-free birth. And the model for new motherhood is a woman who immediately bonds with her newborn, has no difficulties breastfeeding and knows exactly how to interpret every one of her baby's coos and cries. During the first few months postpartum, the perfect new mom nurtures her child in such a way that he is the first kid on the block to roll over, walk, talk and hum along with Bach's *Prelude in D Minor*. This accomplishment-focused mother is so busy trying to achieve what she considers to be the essential goals of motherhood, that it is no wonder she is left with no time to contemplate what being a mother means in the context of her own personal universe. And that self-analysis can be crucial as a woman attempts to navigate the postpartum period and life with an infant.

Throughout the transition to motherhood, a woman may ponder the question "Who am I?" as she tries to incorporate the unfamiliar role of mother into her identity. An expectant mother's changing view of herself is just one of the many things that can affect her adjustment during this transition. Others include the degree to which she desires to become a mom, her earliest childhood experiences with her own mother, her general reflections of family life, and her relationship with her husband or partner. The extent to which she buys into societal expectations regarding motherhood also influences how she will experience the shift to her colossal new role.

Am I ready to be a mother?

The middle name Wande chose for her daughter, England, is *Omotanwa*, a Nigerian word meaning "the child we have been expecting, the one we have been waiting for." Wande believes the years she spent waiting to have a child helped prepare her for motherhood. She had an abortion about a year after she and her husband, Dino, started dating. Later, they had difficulty getting pregnant. "We said, 'OK, well maybe since the abortion, God's punishing us by not granting us a child,'" she recalls. Wande eventually became pregnant but suffered a miscarriage. "So we said, 'OK, God's punishing us again. But maybe he's just trying to prepare us for parenthood.' And that's why once I had the abortion, and then once we had the miscarriage, I said, 'OK, this is it. We have to get ourselves together.' So then I was ready mentally," she declares. Asked what she and Dino had to do in order to "get themselves together," Wande answered, "You can't be booming music in the back of your truck like you used to. You have to make some lifestyle changes and habit changes." Wande, whose husband, Dino, is in the entertainment business and spends a fair amount of time promoting events at nightclubs, says those lifestyle changes meant not "keeping company" with people who were "wild or sleazy." Five years after the abortion, they had the baby they had been waiting for.

First-time mothers give birth to 40% of the children born in the United States each year.[17–19] These women head into labor and delivery rooms with varying degrees of readiness for motherhood. Some pregnant women charge right in. Before the birth of her twins, Shayna, from Virginia, said, "I can't wait to meet them, I can't wait to hold them. Seeing Kevin with a baby yesterday, it was like, 'They're going to give *me* two of these, and I get to take them home, and they're going to be mine. I can't wait to give them everything they need.'" But others head to the finish line with a little less gusto. And then there are women who believe that no amount of preparation can adequately prepare them for what lies ahead.

It is impossible to predict all the changes that will occur during the transition to motherhood; nevertheless, it is important for an expectant mother to be able to acknowledge that life after birth will not simply mirror her pre-baby existence with a child penciled into the picture. These changes will not necessarily have a negative impact on her life. Nor do they mean that she will never enjoy aspects of her pre-baby life. However, the changes do guarantee one thing: a new mother's life will be inevitably transformed. Three-and-a half months before her daughter was born, Kelly said that although she wanted to become a mom, she worried her new role might eclipse the rest of her identity. "Intellectually, I know that change is necessary. Some of the biggest changes I've made were some of the best things I ever did, and I'm grateful for that. This is bigger than anything I could ever dream of. So I'm hoping that I fall so in love with this baby, that it won't matter that I feel like crap or it won't matter that it hurts to breastfeed or that I haven't brushed my teeth. ... I don't want to lose my sense of self. That's my biggest fear. ... If you lose your sense of self, you might as well be dead inside," she declares.

Harriet Lerner, a psychologist and the author of *The Mother Dance: How Children Change Your Life*,[20] writes that even when a woman's pregnancy goes well, it is still a lesson in "surrender and vulnerability." She continues, "No matter how well you prepare yourself, you are not going to be able to run the show. You're in the thick of a full catastrophe, and change is the only thing you can count on for sure."[20]

A little anxiety is perfectly normal as an expectant mother segues into this new phase of her life. Just hours before giving birth, Maggie said, "If we waited another two years, I don't think we'd be any more ready." And a few months before her own delivery, Jodi joked, "I would love to postpone the birth. Am I really ready for this? I think the only thing I'm apprehensive about is: Where do I stand as a human being after this happens as a woman?"

Mothers and daughters

Pregnancy and birth can trigger a flood of memories for an expectant mother about her own upbringing and, in the process, reveal a wealth of information about her relationship with her own mother. All of a sudden, a woman may recall how supportive her own mother was, what her mother sacrificed for her, or how her mom attended every one of her sporting events. A new or expectant mother may also face painful or sad memories, instances when her own mom somehow failed her, constantly criticized her or disappointed her. A woman uses these experiences, both positive and negative, to start to define what type of mother she would like to be. She determines how she wants to be like her own mother and how she would like to be different. This evaluation becomes part of the foundation for her ideas about motherhood.

Minnesota mom LeeRan has always been very close to her own mother, apart from one rough patch. Her mother was a single mom for most of LeeRan's childhood, divorcing her father when LeeRan was three and not marrying again until LeeRan was 15. LeeRan says her mother did the best that she could parenting solo, and tried to be involved in her and her siblings' lives. "When we got sick, she would leave work. ... She never missed plays. She never missed concerts," LeeRan notes, adding that before her mother left in the mornings, she would always pack their lunches. "Everything appeared to be in order. But it wasn't."

LeeRan says discipline and boundaries were sorely lacking. She describes what life was like as her mother was busy studying for a master's degree and a Ph.D., in addition to working as a high-school math teacher: "We were home alone a lot ... getting into trouble. ... Oh my gosh. We would take out the car when she wasn't using it. We'd throw parties. This was when we were a little older. Smoking, drinking, we did it all. I did. My brother and sister not so much, but I was more – I wouldn't say the troublemaker – but I definitely went out and experienced more things, you know, had boyfriends at a young age." LeeRan says she was sexually active by the time she was 15. "Now I look back on that and I'm like, 'That's disgusting. That's out of control. That's so young.' But, you know, we were just so independent and did what we wanted to." LeeRan plans to lay down the law with her son, Matthew. "I think being a good parent is about being able to discipline your child and then walk away from that and not feel guilty about it. And hold your ground."

Thirty-three-year-old Chicago mother Stacey knows she wants to give her daughter, Lainey, the same unconditional love and support that she received from her own mother. "I always felt secure growing up. I always felt loved and cared for. My mom was basically a stay-at-home mom. She worked a couple of days a week at a party goods store. I think that was when I was a little bit older, but she was pretty much a stay-at-home mom. She was there when I got home from school. She was just always there for me. She always gave her attention to my sister and me. We always felt like we came first."

Wande admits that she would be willing to practice tough love just like her own mother did when Wande was a teenager. But Wande vows she will never hit her daughter. She says her mother used to give her what she affectionately calls "whoopin's" whenever she really misbehaved. "I was Satan's child for Christ's sake. Honestly, I don't even know how else to say it. I made her feel guilty about everything. I was very rebellious. I used to sneak out of the house to go out with boys," confesses Wande. Her mother once let her spend the night in jail after Wande had some minor trouble with the police. "I remember her crying as they were taking me to jail because she didn't want to [let them] do it. But I think that's what changed my life right there. Had she not done it, I don't think I would be okay right now. That one day in jail changed my life."

It is not uncommon for a woman whose mother caused her great pain or unhappiness during childhood to want to spare her own children from suffering a similar fate. Becoming a new mom is a chance to start anew, to parent differently in order to avoid making the same mistakes she believes her own mother made. Thirty-eight-year-old Jodi grew up in particularly difficult circumstances. Her mother had multiple sclerosis and was an alcoholic. "My child will never have to put a drunken mother to bed and will not have to be in charge of the family stuff," pledges Jodi. She became the family caretaker because her father – who she says was absent both emotionally and physically – never stepped in to fill that role. "My mother was there physically and she tried to be there emotionally as best as she could, but she just couldn't be there in a supportive way, an encouraging way, a loving way. I mean she couldn't say, 'I think you're wonderful, no matter what! I think you're beautiful, no matter what.'" Jodi says seeking emotional support from her mother was a lost cause. "It was like going to a hardware store for eggs. If I was going to try to get love and compassion from her, it was the wrong place to go."

Jodi remembers that her mother never seemed to provide adequate comfort after typical childhood disappointments, such as the time Jodi failed to become captain of her high-school dance squad. Her mother would make inappropriate comments about the source of Jodi's distress, rather than try to soothe her. "Her response was never, 'That's OK, honey, we love you. It's all right.' It was always like, 'Damn those people, that damn principal screwed you again.' It was never acknowledging, 'I'm really sad that you're sad right now,'" she explains. Jodi says that when her daughter, Tess, is older and experiences disappointment, she will console her and tell her, "'I'm really sorry. I know how painful that must be. I know how much you wanted that.' I want to respect her feelings."

Jodi understood that before she could become a mom, she needed to accept that she would never have a close, supportive relationship with her own mother. "I couldn't bring a child into this world if I hadn't cleared up things in my own life." Implicit in her resolution was that she develop a sense of empathy for the struggles her mother had endured. So after her mom had a stroke, Jodi resolved to accept her mother's shortcomings as a parent, however much pain her mom had caused her, so that she would be able to move forward. Using a common therapeutic technique called visualization, Jodi thought about what she might say to her mom if she knew her mother was going to die. "I got to say to her everything that I wanted to say. I thanked her for everything that she did for me. And I know that she did the best that she could. ... Knowing that she will never be the woman that I want her to be, I have detached myself for the past few years and have taken care of myself."

When a woman analyzes the various dimensions of the relationship she has with her own mother, she can begin to determine what kind of mother she would like to be. Deliberately selecting parenting behaviors is what is called "intentional parenting." A mother (or father) who has not given any thought to how she will parent, may simply resort to "default models" of parenting – provided by her own parents – when she becomes anxious or overwhelmed in her new role. In other words, she will go with what she knows. She may inadvertently adopt her mother's model of parenting, even if she believes that the approach was not particularly helpful to her as a child.[21] Many new mothers are stunned when they find themselves speaking to their children in ways they swore they never would. Some discover that they even inadvertently borrow words and phrases which they loathed hearing in childhood from their own mothers.

Fathers and daughters

There is a reason why so many men cry at their daughters' weddings. A daughter's marriage signifies that her father is no longer the central male figure in her world. Gone are the days when she was a pig-tailed little girl who would sit contentedly nestled in his lap for hours, giggle at all his jokes – even the ones that weren't funny – and practice waltzing across the living-room by standing on his feet. Maybe that is why they have one last dance together at the wedding reception before he sends her off on her new life – to remind her where she has been and where she is going.

Both a father and a mother can offer a daughter guidance, support and unconditional love. But the distinctiveness of the father–daughter relationship is based on what a girl learns about herself through the eyes of a man and what she learns about men in general. In her book, *Women and Their Fathers: The Sexual and Romantic Impact of the First Man in your Life*,[22] researcher Victoria Secunda writes about fathers' "unique value" to girls. She discusses how a father can provide his daughter with, among other things, a "haven" from her mother, plus one man's perspective, validation and affection. Secunda says when a daughter does not have this support and insight from her father, she "aches with questions" and has "no dress rehearsals for heterosexual friendship and love." And she notes that when a woman does not have a father's "dependable involvement" in her life, she "is in some way forever incomplete."[22]

A daughter's relationship with her father enables her to gain another perspective on the differences between femininity and masculinity. Hope Edelman, author of *Motherless Daughters: The Legacy of Loss*, writes, "A father is a daughter's first heterosexual interest, and her relationship with him becomes the most influential blueprint for her later attachments to men."[23] The nature and quality of a daughter's emotional connection with this first love lay the framework for romantic relationships with men throughout her life.

Janine, mother of 5-month-old Nathan, says, "I remember I was 16, and I wanted to drive someplace for a party, and my dad and I got into a fight." Looking back, she suspects he was worried about underage drinking at the party and about drunk drivers. "He came out and said, 'I don't want you to go because I love you.' And that was the first time I ever remember him telling me he loved me." She says that because affection was not something she often saw growing up, "I didn't exactly know what love was. You're just like, 'OK, someone's really nice to me so they must love me.'" Janine continues, "I just want Nathan to know constantly that I love him. I will not only say it but show it as well."

Shayna's father walked out on the family when she was still a baby. As the Virginia wedding coordinator began to think about finding someone with whom she could start her own family, her father's early abandonment was never far from her mind. "I had always wanted to be a mom," explains Shayna. "Having grown up without a father, it was important to me that I trusted the person not to leave."

Vanessa, Virginia mother of 2½-month-old Giavanna, says her own father "loved life" and treated every night as an occasion to celebrate his family. "He'd be home by 4 p.m. He'd put his salsa music on. He would get his glass of wine and he would cook. And my mom would come home at 6:30, and there would be dinner on the table, Monday through Thursday." Vanessa says she loved to watch her parents interact. "I think the most important thing a father can do for his children is to love their mother," she notes. "My dad was so romantic with my mom. He would always buy her flowers. They would always go out to dinner. They were in love until the end. And every time I would look at my father and my mother, I'd be like, 'That's the kind of relationship I want to have, and I'm not settling for anything else.' And I would always tell my dad, 'If I find someone like you, I'm going to marry him.'" A year after her father died, Vanessa went on her first date with Ralph, her future husband. "It was weird. It was like my father sent him down [from heaven]."

A daughter becomes a mother

As a daughter becomes a mother, she may find herself caught between these two roles. A woman, especially after she is married, often feels a need to see herself as independent from her "childhood family." This desire for a sense of autonomy becomes more pronounced once she is pregnant and getting ready to care for her own child. Yet, while she prepares for motherhood, she goes through a period in her life that is physically and emotionally draining, a period during which she herself needs to be mothered.[24] Moreover, as a novice in the parenting world, she will probably turn to someone she knows and trusts for advice – very likely her own mother. So, although she wants to break away from her mother, she would also like her standing by in the wings, ready to swoop in with guidance, a gentle touch and a desire to baby-sit.

The transition to motherhood can help a woman more fully appreciate her own mother's experiences as a parent. Catherine, mother of 5-week-old Matthew, explains that becoming a mom gave her and her mother a new understanding of each other. "She sent me a Mother's Day card this year. It said, 'Welcome to the club.' So I think you relate to each other through an unspoken bond."

Having a baby can serve as a catalyst for reconciliation and can create an opportunity for a parent and child to confront old issues. For Janine, pregnancy and then the birth of her son, Nathan, provided a chance to connect with her mother after years of distance. "It's kind of funny," she says, "I talk to my mother a lot, but I'm not very close to her. I feel like I don't know her that well. But becoming pregnant gave us something in common, and so I feel like we talk more." Janine admits, "I have to say, I now know, because I have Nathan, I understand that my parents did love me. How could you not love your child?" She particularly enjoys watching her mother shower Nathan with affection, and she calls their closeness "amazing" since she does not remember such open displays of warmth and love in her childhood household.

But despite this new mother–daughter closeness, Janine still notices remnants of the childhood relationship she had with her mom. Growing up, Janine was labeled "the athletic one," while her brother was labeled "the intelligent one." And she says not being anointed the smart and talented child undermined her confidence. "I still feel like I can't do anything right in my mother's eyes," remarks Janine. She says that when they visit each other, "I always feel like I'm doing something wrong. A lot of what I do is corrected, or there is a comment about it."

The "good enough" mother

The concept of the "perfect mom," as well as its more recent, trendy incarnations – the alpha mom, the über mom, the supermom – has given mothers a lot to feel guilty about. The pressure to live up to this ideal has mothers constantly assessing their own parenting abilities. In a 2006 *ABC News Good Morning America/Good Housekeeping* poll, 62% of women said they worried about "not being as good a mother as [they] would like to be."[25] Even though plenty of mothers are aware that the perfect mom does not truly exist, this recognition does not stop them from trying to be one. "I think it's important to hold yourself to that high standard though," remarks Jennifer, a Dallas mother of twins. "You've got to put the bar up there. And I do. I think I have unrealistic expectations of myself. But I try so hard because this is just the most important thing I've ever done and I realize that. That's overwhelming, knowing that you're responsible for raising this little life." Jennifer describes the "unrealistic expectations" she had during the first few months postpartum: "I wanted to be there for them all the time even though I was completely exhausted. I wanted to be the one to feed them, bathe them, dress them – *every time*. I wanted to be the one to greet them each morning and put them down each night. That is overwhelming with one baby, much less two! I didn't accept help very well because I thought, as their mother, everything was up to me. I didn't want to let them down."

Sharon Hays, a sociology professor at the University of Southern California, writes about a concept she calls "intensive mothering." She says, "In a society where over half of all mothers with young children are now working outside of the home, one might well wonder why our culture pressures women to dedicate so much of themselves to child rearing." Hays continues,

"In a society where the logic of self-interested gain seems to guide behavior in so many spheres of life, one might further wonder why a logic of unselfish nurturing guides the behavior of mothers. These two puzzling phenomena make up what I call the cultural contradictions of contemporary motherhood."[26]

Although so many women aim to be perfect mothers, they, as well as their children, might be better off if they lowered the bar. Renowned British pediatrician and psychoanalyst D.W. Winnicott coined the phrase "good enough mother." The good enough mother gives to her infant adequate amounts of love and attention in order to meet his psychological needs after he is first born.[27] If we extend Winnicott's "good enough" standard beyond the initial attachment period and apply it to other mothers, not just those of infants, we provide women with an infinitely more realistic goal for motherhood. Good enough mothers properly meet the needs of their children without sacrificing all that is important to them as individuals. This frees up mothers so they are not, as Judith Warner writes in *Perfect Madness: Motherhood in the Age of Anxiety*, "so depleted that we have little of ourselves left for ourselves."[28] Ironically, when a woman strives to be a good enough mother, rather than straining to be a perfect one, she is probably a better parent in the end, since she is not preoccupied with trying to achieve an unattainable ideal. She has more time and energy to concentrate on herself and her own needs. And in the end, that makes her more emotionally available for her children. The oft-quoted mantra bears repeating: A happy mom is a better mom.

Speaking almost a year and a half after her twins were born, Jennifer admits, "I am realizing [motherhood] isn't a sprint, but a marathon. And I am trying to pace myself by taking an hour or two for myself on weekends. I just love being with them and watching them grow and learn, but I need some time to relax and recharge."

What's my role as a mother?

Fifty years ago, the answer was obvious. A mother was the nurturer, caregiver and homemaker, while the father was the breadwinner, moral instructor and disciplinarian. But, those conventional lines have been blurred as more mothers opt to continue working outside the home, and an increasing number of fathers choose to become more intimately involved in the daily lives of their children. Almost every parent interviewed for this book said it is the job of both parents to "always be there" for their children and to provide unconditional love and support. Many of the parents did not differentiate between the roles of a mother and a father, describing similar responsibilities for each. When asked to explain what makes a good mother, Catherine said, "It's hard for me to think about being a mother as being different from being a parent. I see being a parent as being a coach, someone who is going to groom this person and gear him up for adulthood. And that's my job. Now I do think that as a mother ... I want to be a good role model as a female. As a woman, I want to teach my son how to treat women and what women are capable of. I'm very do-it-yourself, home improvement. But at the same time, I can put on a dress and look nice and care about those things."

New York mom Jenny says a good mother "gives children guidance but lets them fail and fall." She explains, "If they never learn how to fail or fall, they're always going to expect everything to be correct, and once they go out on their own, they're going to be extremely disappointed and not realize that that's part of life and growing up." She says children need to learn, from an early age, that everything does not always work out as they hope it will. A child whose parents are always "fixing" imperfect situations for him is not learning how to cope when something does go wrong. So when he is finally on his own, he will have neither the confidence nor the ability to deal with his problems.

Finding role models

Today fictional television role models from the 1950s and 1960s, such as June Cleaver (in *Leave it to Beaver*) and Harriet Nelson (in *Ozzie and Harriet*), seem as outdated as the poodle skirts and saddle shoes so popular when those shows were first aired. Although 5.6 million women in the United States are now stay-at-home moms,[29] they have something the real-life counterparts of June and Harriet did not have – choices. Many of today's new mothers grew up on a steady diet of popular shows featuring working moms – Elyse Keaton on *Family Ties*, the blue-collar Roseanne on the show that bore her name, and of course Clair Huxtable on *The Cosby Show*. Viewers adored Huxtable (played by Phylicia Rashad), an attorney who balanced her responsibilities as a mother, wife and professional with moxie, aplomb and an impeccable wardrobe opposite television's funniest dad.

Both fictional and real-life role models, including a woman's own parents, a favorite aunt, a beloved teacher, influence the kind of mother that a woman chooses to become. Shannon, a 36-year-old mom from Boston, always had unyielding support from her parents. "The best thing that they did was to always make me feel so valued. I never felt like there was anything that I couldn't do. ... And I still to this day feel like if I wanted to run off and be President of the United States, I could do that."

Janine says her mother and father were "functional" but didn't quite measure up in the parenting department. So she "clung" to her best friends and their families, and always had a place at their dinner tables. "I really think that I branched out and took a little bit from my friends and their families," notes Janine. "I noticed that I had friends whose families were very loving and very affectionate."

Jenny views her in-laws as role models. "I want to raise my child the way my husband was raised. His parents were so involved in everything. They guided him without restricting him." She says her in-laws were the kind of parents in whom a child would feel comfortable confiding. "I know your children will hide things from you. But I hope that by bringing up my children the way that my husband was raised, they won't be afraid to come and tell me anything. And if they messed up, they messed up. That's part of life."

Who am I?

Today mothers who were taught that they could have it all – motherhood *and* a successful career – are not sure they even want it all. Some women do, but others are willing to take a pass. In 2004, 55% of women with infants were part of the U.S. labor force, compared with 31% back in 1976, the year the U.S. Census Bureau first started collecting this information.[30,31] In the United states, 70% of mothers with children under 18 years old work outside the home.[32]

These days new mothers have plenty of choices when it comes to combining careers and parenting – part-time, flex-time, job sharing and telecommuting. Ironically, however, all these options have created more dilemmas. A woman trying to sort out who she is, what she wants and what her priorities are may find that her head and her heart are telling her two different things. She may appreciate the sense of accomplishment her career has given her but feel an emotional pull toward her child at home. With each of a woman's roles comes a distinct and sometimes competing set of expectations and responsibilities. And so she may be left asking herself, "Who am I? Who am I to others? What do I expect of myself? What do others expect of me?"

Shannon is a Senior Project Manager for a major financial services firm in Boston. At the time of her interview, she was working part-time, putting in two full days at the office as well as some time at home each week. "In the beginning," the mother of twins says, "I felt like I wasn't doing anything well. I wasn't doing momhood well. I was not doing work well. But now I've kind of reconciled that I'm doing both fairly decently, and that's OK." Doing a good job, rather than a perfect one, can ease the pressure to be everything to everyone at all times. But there are consequences one must accept. "I worked on a project for two years, and it was implemented while I was on maternity leave. And the two people I worked with got promoted, but not me, which was really hard," explains Shannon. "They got promoted for the long hours they put in. Well, I didn't put in those long hours because I wasn't there, but I did work on the project for two years. It's hard. I have to keep reminding myself that if I was working full-time, I literally would see the boys for a half hour in the morning and a half hour at night, if I was lucky. And I can't imagine doing that."

Jennifer works full-time from home as a software implementation consultant. Her twins are never more than a few feet away, unless she is on one of her occasional business trips. But of balancing her roles as a mother and a professional, she confesses, "It's horrible. I hate it. I really do. But that's me. I certainly don't think there's anything wrong with working mothers. That's not at all what I'm saying. I'm just being selfish. I know that this time goes by so fast, and I have always wanted to be a mommy, so I wish I could spend more time doing that." Even though she is the family breadwinner, Jennifer says she views herself as a mother, first. "I feel like this is what I was put on earth for. And I did not know I would feel that way. I really didn't. I mean my first business trip after having them was in May, and I thought I was going to quit my job over it. I mean I was a nut-case ... I enjoy working, and I believe that people should be more than one-dimensional. But frankly, right now I'm really struggling with that because I am one-dimensional."

Maggie, a mother from New Jersey, missed work so much that she cut her maternity leave short in order to return to her job in communications at one of the country's biggest pharmaceutical companies. "I was getting bored at home and needed the structure in my life of returning to work. I wasn't happy and was driving my husband crazy. I didn't know how to stimulate Healey and play with her for 12 hours a day. I'm so glad I did go back. Not only am I happier, but Healey seems happier in daycare five days a week. She loves being with other kids and is learning more than if she were at home with just me all week." Maggie also says her work is an integral part of her identity. "It's something I own, something I'm in control of, the feeling of accomplishment."

After she had her daughter, Lainey, Stacey opted out of the workforce. She had spent a decade in public relations. "I never thought of myself as this career woman. That's just not how I defined myself. So I am happy that I had a really successful, great 10 years, met a lot of great people, was well respected and well thought of – I think so – and now this is my new life. And this is a different stage for me. And I know it won't be like this forever. She's not going to be a baby forever. So at some point, maybe I will go back to working part-time or freelancing." Stacey admits that there are times when she misses the outside world of work. "I love Lainey and would never change a thing. I really do enjoy being home with her like 95% of the time. But I definitely do miss getting up in the morning and having a purpose, you know, showering, getting dressed, putting on make-up and getting out the door at 7:30, 8 o'clock to go to work." Stacey also misses the social component of the work environment, which includes "being with adults all day and being a little more mentally stimulated."

Our identities in the workplace are shaped by external feedback in the form of performance reviews, raises, promotions and, sometimes, even awards. When women become mothers, they do not get those same kinds of rewards and evaluations at home. Catherine decided to leave her television job to stay at home with her son, Matthew. She found it confusing to operate without the same measures of success she had in the business world. "You don't have the same things by which to measure yourself as you did before, like, 'Oh, you did a really good job,' 'Oh, you're making more money at this,' or 'You're going on an exciting trip for work.'" So Catherine has learned to assess her success as a mother in different terms. She explains, "I measure myself by how well it's going and how well my son is doing. And when I go out in the world and everyone tells me, 'Oh, he's so happy, he's so healthy and beautiful,' I just think, 'Well, I'm doing great.'"

CHAPTER 4

Fatherhood: the psychological experience

There was a time when a chapter about an expectant father's psychological experience would not have had a place in a book about pregnancy and parenthood. Ever the detached and sedate financial provider, a man was not supposed to talk about his emotional state or acknowledge his feelings, especially when they concerned subjects such as pregnancy and birth, long considered a woman's domain. His job was to get the process started and then to support his wife. However, a man's emotional experience during the transition to parenthood is far more significant than previous generations realized.

Just like his pregnant partner, an expectant father faces a whirlwind of uncertainty, doubt and introspection. Although he does not undergo any physical changes during the pregnancy (other than perhaps a sympathy weight gain), the prospect of becoming a parent changes the way he views himself, his partner and his responsibilities. And because of social stigmas about men expressing their emotions, the expectant father often must walk the road to parenthood alone, in silence. But, beneath that façade of silence, expectant fathers have a lot to say about their journeys to parenthood.

Am I ready to be a father?

There is no set timetable for "parenthood readiness." Everyone moves at his own individual pace. This was especially apparent when the expectant and new fathers interviewed for this book discussed whether they were emotionally prepared to welcome their children into the world. Some declared that they had been ready since the day they met their wives, or even earlier. Others were in the same camp as 34-year-old father Dino, who asserts "I don't think anyone can ever be ready."

For some fathers, the "right time" means they have built up all the necessary kid credentials: They are financially stable, established in a career and have a house with enough space. Yet, psychologically, they might be wavering, especially if they have acquiesced to a partner's desire to have children. One of life's great paradoxes is that we often desire something more once we find we cannot have or attain it. Chicago attorney Loren always liked children: "I was a camp counselor for many years when I was in college, and I always liked working with children and being around children. I have to say that I always thought that I would have children, but I didn't have a burning desire to have them." It ended up taking Loren and Stacey a year to conceive. Those 12 months of waiting "definitely increased the anticipation and excitement, which was good," notes Loren. "I think maybe it helped us become more ready to be parents because we just wanted it that much more. It actually turned out to be a good thing for us."

Like father, like son?

Even as young children, we begin to note how responsive, reliable and available our parents are as caregivers. As we move toward adulthood, these recollections help us determine the kind of parents we want to be. We sort through these memories to figure out which aspects of our own mother's and father's parenting styles we would like to emulate, and which we would like to avoid. It has been suggested that in order for a man to create his own identity as a father, he identifies certain behaviors "as conforming to 'good' or 'bad' father types."[33]

Ralph remembers that his parents always made their children a priority. Although his father was busy working his way up the ranks of the army to become a two-star general, Ralph's dad still had plenty of time to spend with him and his four siblings. "He traveled a lot, but he coached all of us in sports. So he was very involved and always a very wise person to go to for advice." But, Ralph says, "I'd like to spend even more time with my family, and I think nowadays that's even more important. Possibly down the road, I'd like to have something where I'm working out of the house or owning a business where I could spend as much time as I wanted to with my family."

Kevin wants to show his twins, Hayden and Sydney, the same kind of loving support his father managed to give him, even as his father faced tremendous adversity. His dad endured numerous hardships after injuring his back in a logging accident. Physically unable to continue working as a logger, he was forced to take a job as a security guard, which "he hated." He later developed heart disease and eventually lung cancer. "He did really care. That is the thing that came through," says Kevin. I think he truly cared, which I can't always necessarily say about my mother. ... If I needed something emotionally, I could go to [him]."

Kevin's dad planned special father–son excursions so they could spend time getting to know each other. Kevin (evidently an animal lover) appreciated the effort and interest but not his father's choice of bonding activities. "He took me fishing, which I think is awfully barbaric. And he showed me how to catch a frog, which is even more barbaric," remembers Kevin.

Memories like these can crop up at any point along the journey to parenthood. Bryan says his wife's pregnancy triggered painful memories of his relationship with his father, whom he describes as emotionally detached and unsupportive. He admits, "I feel resentful of my father and have spent most of my days during this pregnancy deciding to do the exact opposite of whatever he did. I'm scared about repeating the mistakes that my dad made, and am so afraid that my kids will think about me the way I think about my dad. I felt like a nuisance. My father was always preoccupied. I wish that he could have been a listener, instead of a lecturer. I want to be able to understand my child's experience."

So strong were Bryan's feelings about his own father that they invaded his dreams. During his wife's pregnancy, his dreams reflected both a longing for a special connection with his unborn child and a terrible fear that his son would rebuff him as he had rebuffed his own father. "I dreamed that the baby was talking to me at the delivery and told me to 'go away and leave him alone.'"

David, an actor who specializes in voiceover work, also wants to be a very different type of father than his own dad was when David was growing up. His father worked hard to provide for the family, putting in 70-hour weeks as an ophthalmologist. David says his father was so focused on work and on making enough money to support the family, that he was frequently absent both physically and emotionally. David has very few memories of special times spent with him. "One was kicking a ball in the backyard, and one was playing basketball. But we weren't really playing; I was just shooting hoops, getting the rebounds, and he was throwing them back to me." The cumulative experience of their father–son ski outings could serve as an appropriate metaphor for their relationship. "I can't remember ever going down the same slope. I don't remember going up the lift together. We did nothing together."

David, who was interviewed before the birth of his daughter, Tess, and then afterward, says he wants to connect with his daughter in a way that he never did with his own father. For him, family life means togetherness and a place where laughter presides. Given the flexibility of his schedule, David spends a good portion of each day with Tess. It is the little things he does with her, such as going to the swings in the park, sharing corned-beef sandwiches at the local deli (when she was old enough to eat them) and window shopping at the mall, which he enjoys most. Even as David tries to build his acting career, he has made spending time with his daughter a priority. He has even found a way to integrate her into his work life. Better than any entourage, Tess has become his little Hollywood sidekick. David says, "Every day I hang out with her. She comes with me to everything. I've had producers holding her while I'm in the [voiceover] booth. ... She comes to my auditions." And he laughs, "We've been to my agent's [office] literally 70 to 80 times. My agents don't even want me in their office without her."

Thirty-four-year-old Cleveland dad, Brett, is determined to be more patient than his own father was. "I think back to my dad who passed away when I was nine. He was a pretty short-tempered guy, and so that's certainly something I need to address and change about myself." He adds, "I don't want to be short-tempered and show [my son] too much anger. And my wife points that out to me very well. She says, 'Watch out because he's watching you. So when he's 2-years-old throwing a temper tantrum, don't get upset with him because he's learning it from you right now.' That's a great point she makes," concedes Brett.

Other role models

While many men view their own fathers, and mothers, as parental role models, others will discover that they need to look beyond their own families in order to find a suitable example of what it means to be a good father. Jim's childhood was defined by poverty, in addition to physical, verbal and emotional abuse, constant moves from state to state, and even an eviction from a housing project. Jim's father abandoned the family when Jim was 4 years old. His mother quickly married another man who physically abused Jim and his siblings. "We joke about it now," says Jim, "but I used to sleep with a baseball bat under my bed." Jim also talks about how his mother abused them. "Her favorite form of torture was – this one's a little tough for me to face – if we would act up or speak out, if we stepped out of line, she would literally bring us to the kitchen and fill our mouths with dish soap." Forced to swallow the soap or, in some instances, Tabasco sauce, they were sometimes so sick they would have to miss school for days. Jim refers to her disciplinary tactics as "crazy little tortures."

When Jim was older, he had to take time off from college to assume legal guardianship of his siblings, apply for public assistance and set up an apartment for the three of them. But, throughout the years, as Jim was managing to keep his little family together, he met two people who showed him what it meant to be a loving and supportive parent. One was the father of his junior high-school friend Steve. "I would sleep over his house for the weekend, so I got a glimpse of what life was really supposed to be like," recalls Jim. "I got to see how a middle-class family lived. ... And we would go on little hikes in the woods together, we'd go canoeing. All of a sudden it was like, 'Wow! Not everybody lives like we do.' It was really eye-opening. And I really started to try to model myself after Steve's father ... and then, after that, George later on in life. So you just start to put the pieces together about what feels good to you as a child or as an adolescent, and then that's how I wanted to be as a father."

George was the stepfather of a girlfriend. Jim calls him "a surrogate father," explaining, "He just took me under his wing. He didn't have any of his own children. We would just go do traditional things like fishing. He had a friend who owned a garage, and we'd go down to the garage and work on the cars and just spend time together, just talking. I only had about six months with him before he passed away from cancer, but he was unbelievable. He made me feel loved and valuable." That is how Jim wants to be with his son, Nathan. "Letting him know that above anything else, I want to spend time with him and share in his life," remarks Jim. Listening to Jim's wife, Janine, it sounds as if he has managed to accomplish this. Janine gushes, "Oh, it's amazing. Regardless of what he grew up with, it's amazing. Just to see Nathan look at him and Jim look at Nathan is so sweet. They have such a great relationship. They have so much fun together. He just makes Nathan scream and laugh. Nathan follows him around the room. When Jim tries to go to the bathroom, Nathan's there, wants to be with him all the time. The older that Nathan gets, the more he's attached to Jim."

Jim's story illustrates how a less than idyllic upbringing does not destine one to repeat history, and how fatherhood is a chance to make a clean start. Having the power to choose what kind of parent one would like to be is sometimes cathartic. It may even help to heal the disappointments of childhood.

Mothers and sons

Ralph's mother had multiple sclerosis and died when he was 16 years old. "She was sick for most of my life, and I think I started noticing it when I was four or five," he recalls. She showed him what it meant to persevere for the sake of family. "My mom was home with five kids while my dad was away at war for two years. ... She'd walk me to school even though she had a tough time walking when I was in first grade. She'd try to drive places though she probably shouldn't have been driving. She'd try to discipline us even though she didn't have the strength to sometimes." Ralph's mother, along with his father, showed him the true meaning of marital commitment. "They lived their vows. They lived the vow of 'in sickness and in health' and they lived the vow of 'No matter what comes our way, we'll stay with each other.'"

Mark describes his mother as the real-life Mrs. Cunningham, better known as "Mrs. C" on the hit television series *Happy Days*. In fact, his friends gave her a similar nickname, calling her "Mrs. B." While their mothers were out working, Mark's friends loved to gather at his house after school because his mom fed them and created a warm and welcoming home. It was this emotional experience of "home" that influenced Mark's ideas about marriage and family. "Part of me still comes from the old school – settle down, get married and raise a family," he says. "I really did want to do it where my wife had the option to be a stay-at-home mom. That was important to me. ... It was my preference because this is what I'm used to. When I came home, my mother was there, and the cooking and just the smell of the food – there was a sense of security and warmth that I felt."

A father may teach his son how to be protective and courageous, how to be a team player and how to face performance fears.[34] But, it is usually the mother who focuses on fostering her son's emotional and interpersonal side, and she can play an important role in helping him navigate the intricacies of relationships.[35] Michael Gurian is the author of *Mothers, Sons & Lovers: How a Man's*

Relationship with His Mother Affects the Rest of His Life.[36] He writes that before a son becomes an adult, he is dependent on his mother for certain "elements of his psychological life." These elements include the development of a healthy communication style, a way of handling conflict, his view of femininity, an emotional language to help him identify and express his feelings, and a "sense of safety in the world."[36] Both Gurian and Jerrold Shapiro, author of *The Measure of a Man: Becoming the Man You Wish Your Father Had Been,* point out that a mother serves a broad but essential role in helping her son figure out just who he is. "The mother plays a very important and powerful role with regard to how he experiences himself as a person. And, of course, that's core for being anything [in life]," says Shapiro, Chairman of the Counseling Psychology department at Santa Clara University.

Although the male figures in his life disappointed him, 35-year-old D.J., an advertising sales manager at a major newspaper, knew he could always count on his mother. The Kentucky dad has no childhood memories of his father, who divorced his mother when D.J. was about three. His mother then married a man who, D.J. says, was the type of parent who "would rather give you $20 and tell you to go buy something for yourself than play ball with you or go to one of your games." D.J. never felt as if he could depend on his stepfather. He recalls one incident in particular. "I was either 8 or 9 and the Harlem Globetrotters were coming to Cincinnati, and I'd been promised all along we were going. It was right around my birthday in February. It was a big deal. I'd been looking forward to it, and when the time came, he had to work late and we didn't end up going. And I remember that night being absolutely crushed and lying in my room and just bawling," says D.J. "I remember just a blatant disregard for what was important to me."

D.J. says he views his mother as a parental role model because she was the one who taught him the meaning of unconditional love. "She was very nurturing. There was never any point – even during that rebellious teenage time when you're mad at your mom – there was never a point when I didn't think that she didn't love her boys as much as she possibly could. Did she make mistakes as a mother? Yes, I think everyone does."

What's my role as a father?

A dad in the 1940s and 1950s was the breadwinner, the moral instructor, the protector and the disciplinarian. It was also his job to teach his sons "manly" things, such as how to throw a football, how to cast a fishing line and how to fix a carburetor. His stature as the family authority figure was the reason so many baby boomers heard their mothers threatening, "Wait until your father gets home!" Television aptly depicted the stereotypical 1950s father with *Father Knows Best*'s Jim Anderson, *Leave it to Beaver*'s Ward Cleaver, and Ozzie of *Ozzie and Harriet*. Today members of the younger generations enjoy lampooning these old favorites that have come to represent such antiquated notions of gender roles.

Men today have more choices and more flexibility in defining their roles within the family. Many fathers spend more time with their children and are more intimately involved in their day-to-day lives. In 1977, men whose wives worked outside the home spent barely two hours each workday with their children. According to the Families and Work Institute's data on men in dual-earner couples, in 2002, fathers spent an average of 2.7 hours per workday with their children.[37] The numbers are even more remarkable for Gen-X dads (fathers aged 23 to 37), who spent 3.4 hours per workday with their kids.[38] Fathers are assuming a greater share of the housework, all the while putting in more hours at work and sacrificing their own free time. In 2002, men (in dual-earner couples) with children had nearly 40% less time for themselves on workdays than their counterparts 25 years earlier.[39]

These days, fathers not only see themselves as providers and protectors, but also as teachers, confidants, playmates, homework helpers, soccer dads and friends. And they are not afraid to get dirty in the trenches changing diapers. Shapiro explains that the women's movement paved the way for fathers to increase their involvement in child-rearing: "As women got more equality in certain ways, it opened it up for men to get more equality in ways for themselves, too. So I think it's been an amazing liberation. ... I think as women became more empowered, they less needed to control the home, and so they opened it up for their husbands to do more. And, of course, some of the husbands raced in there, and some ran to the hills."

Forty-five-year-old Mark "raced in" to share in caring for his newborn son. "I'd like to be close to our son, Matthew, and I'd like to do the things that maybe weren't typical of a father before – feedings, changing diapers, holding him, getting him to relax before bed, walking with him in the middle of the night. I like the idea of doing these things because I think it's going to bring a different type of a bond, an even closer bond than what I have now. I want to feel that I'm able to achieve that by letting him know that I'm there for him in that way," explains Mark.

Mark was also eager to step into a teaching role. "It's something I've always looked forward to ... to give them skills and knowledge, to help them become independent, self-sufficient, good people," he says. Kevin, a Williamsburg father of twins, wants to be the kind of father who "guides his children through the world, helps them figure out who they are and how to do things, keeps them safe, keeps them out of trouble and helps them to make good choices."

Even though many men see themselves as providers, they do not necessarily define their roles based solely on their ability to bring home the bacon. Today dads make time to fry it up in a pan, enjoy a leisurely meal with their kids and then clear the dishes. Nevertheless, money is still a daunting component of the parenting equation. According to the U.S. Department of Agriculture, a middle-income family will spend $250,000 on a child before he turns 18. That

$250,000 does not even include the cost of college. A couple can expect to spend about $12,700 on a first child by the time they celebrate his first birthday.[40]

Throughout his wife's pregnancy, David, an actor, was constantly worried about money. "I want to bust my ass to create a good life for this child so that I can show her what the world is like. I've always heard stories about my grandfather and how he couldn't keep a job. I'm so worried that I'll be like him," he remarks. Although David does not want to struggle financially like his grandfather, he also does not want to be fixated on earning money the way his father was. So he is trying to strike a balance, to achieve job stability – in an industry known for being difficult and fickle – while continuing to be a hands-on father. "We have trouble with finances now. It's the debate we have: Do I go off and do something where I'm spending all day away, or do we tough it out and continue to do what we're doing? At the moment, we're going to continue what we're doing. ... Right now, things [work-wise] are dead. I haven't been this flat broke in a long time, and it definitely brings up a lot of fears," David says, referring back to his grandfather's financial situation.

Dino, a father from Atlanta who runs his own entertainment and promotions company, has also kicked into high-gear provider mode and, like David, has made spending time with his daughter a priority. "I always had ambitions of being a dad and raising my child with things I didn't have as a kid," he acknowledges. When Dino was growing up, money was tight and he was constantly reminded of the realities of his parents' economic situation: "I came from a lower-middle-class family. I'm a musician. I wanted to play an instrument at an early age, but I couldn't do that because my parents couldn't afford it."

Dino wants to ensure that his family can have a more comfortable lifestyle. "I have a very successful business, and I have a wonderful family," he says. "I live in a nice house. I grew up in a small house. I grew up in a three-bedroom house with a brother and a sister. So my brother and I shared a room the whole time. Here, England's not going to have to do that. ... Right now, I'm kind of living my dream." And he is teaching little England a thing or two on the miniature piano he bought for her when she was just 3 months old.

Today's "good father"

Almost every one of the men interviewed for this book defined a good father as one who is emotionally available for his children. They emphasize that a good father is "always there" to comfort his children, to help them make appropriate choices, to instill confidence in them, and to support them in times of trouble. According to D.J., being a good father is about being a good role model: "[It's about] being somebody Cooper can look to and say, if nothing else, 'My dad lives his life the right way. And if I live mine like he does, I'm probably in good shape.' I think the other thing is just being there for him no matter what, you know, supporting him in what he does, supporting him when he's older by giving him some decision-making opportunities. And if he makes bad ones, being there and supporting him and helping him learn from those mistakes."

Ralph, father of 10-week-old Giavanna, says being a good father means always putting the family first. "I think a good father will do everything and anything to keep that priority consistent no matter what situation he faces in life," he states. In order to make his family a priority, Ralph took what he viewed as a less prestigious position at a radio station in Washington, D.C. "I was in management. I actually just changed that, and I jumped back into sales. And the major reason I jumped back into sales was because of my situation with the family ... to give myself a little more flexibility. And it's a position where I can make more money and have more time with my family. It's just less responsibility. It was a shot to the ego, but, once again, it was a decision of keeping the priorities I had established. I'm putting my family first, and this was a wise move for me to make."

Fathers are created, not born

It is one thing for expectant fathers to wax philosophical about fatherhood and all that it entails. It is quite another to be a father once the baby is born. The psychological process of becoming a father does not occur overnight. Scott Coltrane, a sociology professor at the University of California, Riverside, has been studying family and gender issues for 23 years. He notes, "As a culture, we're beginning to understand that parenting is not built into our genes. It's not an automatic response. Women have to learn how to do it just like men have to learn how to do it. It's on-the-job training."

Women may gain some of this experience during adolescence and early adulthood. But, Coltrane says men do not typically get this training until they have kids of their own. "We don't direct our boys into doing a lot of babysitting or caring for kids in the way that we have with girls. And so, generally, women enter relationships where they're going to have kids much better prepared. But once men start to get involved, they learn how to do it just like women do."

An expectant father can use the months before the baby is born to start preparing for the changes and challenges he will soon encounter. It is a time to contemplate the ways in which he and his partner can maintain a satisfying relationship, and how his sense of himself will shift to that of "family man."[41]

Traditionally, in our society, it was regarded as a sign of weakness for a man to talk about his feelings. To some extent, this is still true. But by discussing his psychological experience of impending fatherhood, a father-to-be paves the way for a smoother transition to parenthood, for both himself and his partner. Identifying and discussing concerns can free him up emotionally and mentally so he can focus on the most important tasks at hand: adjusting to fatherhood, supporting his partner, and bonding with and enjoying his new baby.

CHAPTER 5

Labor and delivery

The nine months of waiting, worrying and dreaming have all been leading up to this – the birth, the day when expectant mothers and fathers officially become parents. There is no way to predict exactly what will transpire on an emotional level for a couple as they kick off "Labor Day." Even with a relatively straightforward birth, labor and delivery can be a psychologically complex event. It is a time of great highs and lows. The emotions an expectant couple may experience during childbirth run the gamut – anxiety, relief, anger, joy, embarrassment, helplessness, detachment and even ambivalence. A woman may feel euphoric after learning she is dilated three centimeters, but later feel disappointed or despondent when the birth does not progress as quickly or as easily as she had anticipated. Or a man may feel instant love for his new baby just as he is becoming increasingly apprehensive about the responsibilities that lie ahead. In short, labor and delivery is often a time of emotional overload as future parents head toward the finish line and get ready to assume the biggest roles of their lives.

It does not help that expectant couples tend to arrive at the hospital emotionally encumbered by misconceptions about labor and delivery. The sources of these misguided beliefs? Family members, friends, co-workers, neighbors, even the woman at the supermarket checkout counter. Most of us are only too eager to share dramatic birthing stories about 43-hour labors or hospitals so full that women were delivering their babies in the hallways.

The media also shapes our ideas about the childbirth process. Just as some people are convinced that they will have a horrendous birth experience after hearing their friends' frightening accounts, others are blissfully ignorant, having bought into Hollywood's sanitized and romanticized version of labor and delivery – quick, clean and oozing joy. Catherine contends that, in the movies and on television, they show only "the pushing part." "But it's the hours leading up to it; they don't show the part where you are writhing in pain. Oh my God!" she exclaims.

Expectant parents should bear in mind that each birth is unique, defined by its own distinctive rhythms, intensity of pain, length of labor and delivery, and memorable moments. Although it is natural for parents-to-be to want to gather information about this momentous event, it is important that they carefully filter the steady stream of information flowing their way. They may find it useful to enlist the help of their obstetrician/gynecologist, midwife or childbirth class instructor to assist them in separating fact from fiction. Armed with some helpful, and accurate, background information, they will be in a better position to discern which of these tales have most likely been embellished to enhance their entertainment value at the water cooler, and are, therefore, not a cause for concern.

Expectant parents who approach labor and delivery with realistic expectations, and who understand the possible complications that may occur, can reduce their stress levels and have a more satisfying birthing experience. Educating themselves about the childbirth process can help them maintain some perspective on the big day, when things may not be going according to plan, and anxiety and frustration levels are running high. For example, what does it mean if the cord is wrapped around the baby's neck? Why might doctors need to perform a cesarean section? How does a forceps delivery work? Often there is nothing to be concerned about, scary as situations like these may sound to laypeople.

Finally, expectant parents stand a better chance of weathering the physical and emotional strains of labor and delivery if they arrive at the hospital knowing what they want from the childbirth experience. That they desire a birth in which the health of neither the mother nor the child is compromised is a given. That they would like a quick, complication-free labor and delivery is also understood. But, an expectant mother and father may want to clarify what they expect of each other; what they can reasonably expect of the medical staff regarding care, communication and timely updates; how they might feel about a cesarean section should one be necessary; and what measures the mother would be willing to take to alleviate pain. They may also want to consider even more mundane issues, such as how they might pass the time waiting for their little one to make his or her big debut. In addition, expectant parents will feel more confident and empowered during labor and delivery if they are able to identify and accept that certain aspects of the process are within their control, while others are not. In some instances, fate will trump even the most meticulous planning.

What if ...?

"Since the day we met, since the day we fell in love, and we knew we were meant to be together, I was always terrified of something happening to her during childbirth," says Bryan of his wife, Marla. Asked why he feels this way, the Laguna Beach, California dad responded, "I have absolutely no control over what happens during the birth. And I'm so afraid to lose her because the way I want to have my family includes her. Without her, I don't have a plan."

It comes as no surprise that expectant parents' top fears about labor and delivery concern the well-being of the mother and child. In fact, one study found that two of the most common sources of stress for an expectant father are the baby's condition at birth and his partner's pain during labor and delivery. Far more men were worried about these things than about financial issues related to the addition of a child.[42] Another study cited fear of pain during labor and delivery as among the most frequent causes of stress for women. Physical distress such as fatigue, nausea and vomiting, concerns about body image and concerns about their babies' well-being were also all high on the list.[43]

Vanessa was studying for her nursing degree and working as a clinical technician before she gave birth to her daughter. Despite having a medical background, she still let her imagination get the best of her after speaking with a friend who just had a baby. That friend managed to feed into Vanessa's fears about pain associated with the birthing process. "She said 'Oh my God, Vanessa. It's the worst pain you'll ever go through.' And I'm just like, 'Thanks.'" As a result, Vanessa went into labor and delivery thinking that she would experience the "worst pain."

Jennifer, mother of twin girls, Katy and Ally, remembers, "I was just worried about pain and exhaustion. And what would happen if I had to deliver one vaginally, and then they had to go take the other one via C-section? So I would basically get the worst of both scenarios." Jennifer was especially concerned about labor and delivery *after* having taken birthing classes. "I was a nutcase. I did not want to have a vaginal delivery and I did not want a C-section, so I was out of choices. I was thinking, 'Let's keep them in until they come up with a third way to get these things out.'"

Going into labor and delivery, it is easy to imagine the worst. The logistics alone are frightening. After all, how can it *not* hurt to push a 7-pound baby out of such a normally small opening? "As the days go by, and the baby does get bigger and bigger, it makes me a little more nervous. How am I going to get this baby out?" wonders LeeRan just a few weeks before delivering Matthew.

Even when a woman has had a healthy pregnancy, she and her partner still tend to worry about potential complications during childbirth that could put the baby at risk. "I'm worried that the umbilical cord will be around the baby's neck or that the baby will have fetal distress," says Maggie, shortly before the birth of her daughter. An umbilical cord around the baby's neck is not necessarily a cause for alarm, unless it is wrapped so tightly that it is restricting the flow of blood to the fetus. If that is the case during labor and delivery, the baby can be delivered immediately via a cesarean section or forceps delivery. Expectant parents also tend to worry about the baby having respiratory problems following delivery, or birth defects, including an incorrect number of fingers and toes. (Why else would so many brand-new parents bother to count them!)

Birth plans

A birth plan is a document written during pregnancy which states what the couple expects and wants during labor and delivery. In it, the mother-to-be can note whether she would like an epidural and/or pain medication, whether she would like to be mobile during labor, in which position she would prefer to deliver the baby (i.e. lying down, squatting, sitting) and whether she wants an episiotomy. In this one-page document, a father can express his desire to cut the umbilical cord, and the couple can list who is allowed in the birthing room. This can mean barring entry to a team of eager young medical students or an overbearing mother-in-law. A mother-to-be may want to note whether she would like to hold her baby immediately following delivery, before the child is whisked away to be cleaned up and examined. In addition, a birth plan is a good place for an expectant parent to mention his or her particular fears about labor and delivery, so the medical staff is aware of them before the birth.

This plan helps couples feel as if they have some modicum of control over the birthing process. And it enables the mother-to-be to take charge of what is happening to her own body. In one study, 93% of women said having a birth plan improved their understanding of the choices available to them during labor, 89% stated that it improved their understanding of the options during delivery, and 81% said they became more aware of the alternatives available to them after birth.[44]

But in the heat of the moment, when pain and fear are most likely to cloud thinking, even the best birth plan may go out the window. "It didn't even make it in the house! Just out the window," jokes Wande. "And I really worked hard on that birth plan. I'd say I spent at least a week writing it. I went to all the Internet sites and looked at sample birth plans, went to birth classes and put it together. ... My birth plan said, 'By any means necessary, do not give me an epidural." But sure enough, in the throes of labor, Wande opted for one. A 1998 study published in the journal *Midwifery* found that 60% of women surveyed deviated from their birth plans, although most were not upset about having done so.[45]

Whether expectant parents create a formal written document, or just discuss their expectations for the birth, they should make sure that they review the plan with their midwife or doctor well in advance of the due date. These healthcare providers will be able to tell them which of the requests are realistic, given the hospital's facilities, as well as their own experiences with women in labor and delivery. For example, Kelly's doctor recommended that she be a little more open-minded about medical interventions. "He said, 'Why don't you want [the labor-inducing drug] Pitocin?' And then he said, 'I'm not going to give you anything that you're not going to absolutely need.' So I adjusted the plan to 'No Pitocin unless I absolutely need it, and no epidural unless I request it,'" explains Kelly.

Studying for "labor day"

Childbirth classes can help provide expectant couples with peace of mind by making the unfamiliar somewhat more familiar. Typically, instructors will explain what happens during labor and delivery, how complications are handled, and what types of pain management and coping techniques can be used. They also give tours of the hospitals' birthing facilities. Many mothers- and fathers-to-be enjoy the social aspect of the classes and the chance to commiserate with other first-timers preparing to take the plunge into parenthood. The classes can also make men feel more a part of the birthing experience. Ralph declares, "I think it's better for the men than it is for the women. Generally speaking, women seem to be much more interested, and they read more about what their bodies are going through. ... They seem to get into it more. Men don't seem as interested or at least don't want to act like they are in front of other men." Ralph was so enthusiastic about educating himself, he even went to a breastfeeding class, as did Bryan.

Expectant parents should consider what type of preparation might be most valuable to them in the labor and delivery room. Some people simply want a primer that explains the different stages of labor, the various medical options for relieving pain and a few basic breathing exercises. In contrast, others actively seek out classes that emphasize an "intervention-free" birth. Students in these classes learn how to manage labor pain sans medicine and an epidural, by focusing on the natural rhythms of the body in labor and engaging in mental exercises to release fear.

Childbirth class options include:

- *Lamaze.* This is the "Kleenex" of childbirth classes. Although some people use the word "Lamaze" generically to refer to all childbirth classes, they do not realize that Lamaze represents a specific birthing philosophy. Lamaze stresses natural childbirth, which means "no routine inter- ventions" – including epidurals, electronic fetal monitoring and IVs – unless " medically necessary." The well-known "hee-hoo" breathing exer- cises are no longer Lamaze's hallmark, although instructors do teach breathing techniques, along with other coping strategies. Lamaze endorses continuous labor support. It is important to note that some classes may claim to be "Lamaze-based," meaning they teach some of the Lamaze tech- niques but also review medical options for relieving pain and inducing labor.
- *Bradley Method.* The Bradley Method is an intense 12-week (one 2½-hour class per week) course that goes into extensive detail on nearly every aspect of pregnancy and childbirth. Students even get workbooks. The Bradley Method concentrates on relaxation, exercise and nutrition. Like Lamaze, it emphasizes a natural birth. Husbands (or partners) are expected to take an extremely active coaching role.
- *HypnoBirthing.* This technique was developed by a hypnotherapist in 1989. It teaches women how to "release fears" and relax themselves into a dream- like state in order to alleviate pain and stress.

Two other programs that take an introspective approach to labor and delivery are *Birthing from Within* and *Birth Works.*

Many of the classes offered through hospitals and OB-GYN offices are taught by someone who is a labor-and-delivery nurse and/or certified birth instructor. Lamaze International, the American Academy of Husband-Coached Childbirth (Bradley Method) and organizations such as the Association of Labor Assistants and Childbirth Educators (A.L.A.C.E.) and the Academy of Certified Birth Educators and Labor Support Professionals all certify instructors.

Although some people, like Dallas mother Jennifer, become increasingly apprehensive after taking a childbirth class, others contend that the knowledge they gain boosts their overall psychological comfort level. They may still be anxious, but at least they have a better understanding of what will happen and why.

The birthing partner's role

These days it is hard to imagine a woman giving birth without a friend or relative by her side, supporting her, holding her hand, and wiping her face with a cold washcloth. Not too long ago, labor and delivery rooms were lonely places for pregnant women because hospitals barred their husbands from being present during the birth. Dr. Fernand Lamaze set out to change that.

During the early 1950s, Dr. Lamaze introduced his childbirth techniques in France, borrowing from methods he had observed in Russia. His approach included relaxation, special breathing exercises and constant support from the husband. An American actress named Marjorie Karmel, who had visited Dr. Lamaze when she was in Paris, boasted of his birthing methods in a book entitled *Thank You, Dr. Lamaze*, and created a buzz back in the United States. In 1960, she and Elizabeth Bing formed what would later be known as Lamaze International. Meanwhile, obstetrician Dr. Robert Bradley was busy promoting his natural approach to the birthing process, which also emphasized husband-coached childbirth, and in 1965 he published a book entitled *Husband-Coached Childbirth: The Bradley Method of Natural Childbirth*.

By the 1970s, expectant fathers, previously banished to the waiting room alongside the vending machines, were invited and encouraged to join their partners in the miraculous process of bringing a new life into the world. And today men are *expected* to participate in the birth, even if they are worried about their ability to handle it.

In his 1993 book, *The Measure of a Man: Becoming the Man You Wish Your Father Had Been*, Jerrold Shapiro writes that "85% of all American men in intact families expect to be present at the birth[s] of their children." In the 1960s, that figure was only 15%.[46]

The coach's job is to support the birthing mother in any way possible. This may entail helping her with the breathing exercises, massaging her feet or back, keeping up her spirits, distracting her from agonizing contractions, or offering a silent sign of encouragement by simply holding her hand. In addition, the coach may be in charge of communicating with the medical staff

– getting timely updates on his partner and the progress of the birth, keeping the medical team posted of any changes in her condition and discussing emergency contingencies. However, the coach's main responsibility is to accommodate his wife (or partner) and to make her as comfortable as possible, both physically and emotionally, during labor and delivery.

"I obviously couldn't empathize with the pain Stacey was going through, never having experienced that before. I just wanted to be encouraging and a cheerleader when she needed it, but quiet when she needed that, too," explains Loren, a father from Chicago. One helpful diversion for Loren and Stacey was watching a reality television show. "It was like a normal Wednesday night for us," says Loren.

Ralph drew upon his experience as a college football player during his wife's labor. "I have a big athletic background, so it reminded me of performing for an athletic event. I was really pushing her – not that she needed it – but I was pushing her and doing the countdown, telling her what was left, when to relax, when to go hard. I was just being her little football coach." Ralph says that although they made a great team, his wife, Vanessa, eventually needed a cesarean section.

Jason, a police officer who had been trained to deliver babies, helped his wife, Maggie, with her breathing exercises. As is often the case on the big day, stage fright set in, and Jason could not remember all the specific breathing patterns he and Maggie had learned during their childbirth classes. "I only remembered one of the techniques, so that's the one we used," he recalls. But he did employ another pain coping mechanism from their class – dancing. Although a sterile hospital room would never be confused for *Studio 54*, Jason took Maggie for a little spin across the linoleum tiles. Maggie says, "In our baby class, it was like the eighth-grade slow dance. The woman puts her head on her husband's shoulder. It's supposed to make the contractions feel a little bit better, and it did. It really worked." In addition, Jason brought washcloths and ice chips to make Maggie more comfortable as they waited for their daughter, Healey, to be born.

Dino was the ultimate hands-on coach – he actually helped deliver the baby. He saw how much pain Wande was experiencing and just wanted to help get the baby out so she would feel better. "The doctor was holding the baby's head straight, and I was pulling the body part out. He was stabilizing the head. When she came out all the way, I was holding her in my arms," says Dino. Normally a little squeamish, Dino was too awestruck by the beauty of the delivery to be bothered by its various bodily by-products – blood, mucus, amniotic fluid and the afterbirth. "I was amazed. Just to see her come out and start moving and crying, I was thinking, 'Wow, I can't believe this actually happened.'"

Like Dino, many of the fathers interviewed said they were caught up in the excitement of the moment and did not have time to worry about feeling queasy. Ralph says it was just one of those situations "where you're not even thinking about that stuff. You're doing what's best for your wife and new baby. You're not thinking about being squeamish."

A few of the women interviewed mentioned that they did not want their husbands closely observing "the whole entire thing," as one mother put it. D.J. recalls, "Keri's very self-conscious ... and said, 'I don't want you down there. I want you up by my head.'" For the most part, D.J. complied with Keri's wishes. Only once did he venture down to the opposite end of the hospital bed so the doctor could show him the baby's head.

The coach's performance

Some coaches are helpful, some are helpless and others are a hindrance.

In 2006, Childbirth Connection (formerly known as the Maternity Center Association), an 88-year-old not-for-profit organization dedicated to improving maternity care, published the results of its *Listening to Mothers II* survey. *Listening to Mothers II* is a national survey of more than 1,500 women about their experiences during pregnancy, birth and the postpartum period. The study was conducted in partnership with Lamaze International. In total, 82% of the women surveyed were assisted by their husbands or partners during the birthing process, and 72% of these women gave them an "Excellent" rating in terms of the quality of support they provided. Although only 3% of the women who were surveyed used a doula (a trained labor assistant) during labor and delivery, 88% of these women gave their doulas an "Excellent" rating.[47]

Judith Walzer Leavitt, a professor of history of medicine at the University of Wisconsin and the author of *Brought to Bed: Childbearing in America 1750–1950*,[48] has been studying the history of childbirth for more than 20 years. She says now that men have secured a place in the labor and delivery room: "Some fathers are finding that that role may be helpful to their wives but not helpful to themselves and, therefore, they're voicing some reluctance about going in. I think that still has to do with a question of how much they are educated in what's going to happen, how much they are worried about their own roles and their abilities to take the kind of responsibility that sometimes seems thrust upon them." Leavitt adds that some men "want some space for themselves." They do not want to be "on-duty" for the duration of the labor and delivery. Instead they want the freedom to be able to leave the room for a while to deal with some of the emotions they are experiencing. Fathers-to-be may want to consider hiring a doula or bringing along another birthing partner such as the expectant mom's own mother or a friend.

Roberto and Kelly came fully "staffed" with both his mother and a doula. Speaking before the birth, Roberto noted that although it was comforting to know there would be a professional onboard, he was still scared. "I don't know what I'm going to be dealing with, and I don't know if I'm going to be ready when Kelly freaks out. Whatever I do, it's going to be wrong." As it turns out, there was a lot of tension between Kelly and Roberto during labor and delivery. "He lost patience with me. He'd get frustrated, and I knew he wanted it to be over," states Kelly. "He was pissed that I didn't volunteer and say, 'OK, let's do a C-section now.'" Roberto argues that if Kelly had opted for a cesarean section earlier, she could have spared their baby some of the distress of the lengthy labor. "Since midnight the previous night, her heart rate would drop every once in a while. You have no idea how nerve-racking it is to hear the heartbeat coming out of the machine and actually have the feeling that your baby could die," says Roberto, concluding, "I was very resentful at the time because as the father of the child, I was completely left out [of the decision-making process]. But, of course, everything was fine as soon as Emma was born and she was OK." In hindsight, Roberto realizes that if his daughter's life had truly been in danger, doctors would have performed a cesarean section earlier.

One Finnish study, which tracked fathers' experiences of birth, found that attending the delivery was an important part of men's "growth into fatherhood." The study also revealed that two of the most difficult aspects of labor and delivery for men were feeling helpless and witnessing a wife or partner in pain.[49] New father Mark says, "I had a vision that it was going to be very active and flowing and that we were just going to go through this process, and it just didn't quite go like that. ... At times I was helpless and wasn't able to do what she needed. There were moments when I was dumbfounded. I also felt paralyzed at times." His wife, Catherine expresses her disappointment in Mark's failure to adopt a more "take-charge" attitude: "I was frustrated because at times I felt like, 'Please grab hold of the reins for me because I can't do it right now' ... I would have liked him to be more like, 'OK, let's try this technique, let's do this' ... I felt like I wanted him to look at me and think, 'Oh, she needs me to give her a cold cloth.'"

Considering the potent mix of physical and emotional sensations – anxiety, pain, tension and exhaustion – it is no wonder that more than a few expectant parents have trouble holding their tempers (and their tongues) during labor and delivery. Keri says that D.J. was a terrific coach, yet she found herself losing patience with him, especially before she was given an epidural. "When I was in pain, he would tell me to breathe and to calm down and to explain the pain to him. And I think one time he said, 'It can't hurt that bad.' And I said, 'Nooooooooooo! Get out of here!'" She continues, "I remember before I had the epidural, I was getting angry at him ... just not wanting him to talk to me. I remember just wanting him to be quiet. I think at that time I was blaming him for all of the pain."

Despite tense moments, the shared experience of childbirth can have a positive effect on a couple's relationship.[50] A father who is hesitant about attending the birth should figure out how to address his concerns so he does not have to be absent from what will probably be one of the most profound experiences of his life.

Best laid plans

The coach's performance is only one of many factors that can affect the birthing experience. The length and ease of delivery, the degree to which a couple is accurately informed about the process and, of course, the pain quotient all play important roles. For all the advances in modern medicine, pain is still largely a mystery to scientists. How much discomfort a woman experiences during childbirth may depend on her own individual tolerance for pain, the position of the baby and the amount of preparation she has had. This is not to imply that someone who reads 15 books on childbirth and attends classes religiously will have a pain-free birth. However, a woman who is educated about the birthing process, and who is confident in her ability to use relaxation and pain-relieving techniques, tends to be more comfortable and less stressed, at least during the initial phase of labor.[51]

Twenty-seven-year-old Ginette, from the Bronx in New York, imagined contractions would be painful, but they were far worse than she had anticipated. "I was afraid that each contraction would be longer and more painful. ... The nurse said, 'Breathe, breathe.' I just thought, 'I can't breathe because I just didn't expect it to be that painful!' ... My husband and I had taken several Lamaze classes. We learned the breathing exercises, and we used to practice them at home. But the minute I went into the hospital, I forgot everything."

Ginette is in good company. A lot of people forget the proper breathing patterns on the big day. When push comes to shove, many also question how helpful the exercises really are. In Childbirth Connection's *Listening to Mothers II* survey, 56% of the women who used the breathing exercises described them as "somewhat helpful." Only 21% said they were "very helpful." Not as many women tried the other drug-free, pain-relieving techniques listed in the survey, such as immersion in a tub or pool, the use of a birth ball, and the use of hands-on techniques, including massage and acupressure. But those who did were more likely to rate them as "very helpful."[52]

Wande had assumed she would be able to ride out the pain when she originally opted for a natural birth. "I have a high threshold for pain. I was the queen of pain. But it was crazy," she says of the discomfort she actually experienced. The self-proclaimed queen of pain readily relinquished her throne for an epidural. "I felt like I was being crucified. It was unbearable. I just couldn't take it anymore."

Catherine expected to have a peaceful, quiet birth like the ones she had seen in the videos from her HypnoBirthing class. "I didn't want to go into labor and delivery fearful. I didn't want to go into it with this brace-yourself sort of a feeling. ... Not knowing at all what was going to be, I at least wanted to be relaxed for whatever it was," explains the 40-year-old former television commercial producer. But her serene birth was not to be, and her attempts to eliminate her fears were unsuccessful. "I found it very difficult to relax. I found it difficult to apply the techniques," says Catherine, adding, "I had anxiety in my head about 'How am I going to do this? Am I going to be able to take care of him? Am I going to be able to do it?'"

Many women head for the hospital believing they will deliver exactly the way their own mothers did. Four generations of women in Kate's family gave birth, "from first contraction to delivery," in two hours or less. So Kate naturally assumed she would follow in this tradition. "My mom had me in 55 minutes from first contraction to birth. How mad is that!" she exclaims. "So I was thinking I was in for an easy ride, and I wanted to have either a home birth or a water birth, something relaxed." Relaxed is not the word Kate would use to describe the birth of her son, Elliot. For four days, she and Paul were in labor-and-delivery limbo, with her contractions starting and stopping, then starting again. Her son was finally delivered with a ventouse (a vacuum extraction). Looking back, Kate notes, "It's hard because I did expect a relatively easy labor when I was induced. And I kind of wish I had gone into it thinking, 'This could be a day or two.'"

The notion that a woman's labor and delivery experience will be similar to that of her mother is not just an old wives' tale. But a woman should not rely on her mother's birthing experience as a firm predictor of what her own experience will be like. Dr. Iffath Hoskins, Chairman of the Department of Obstetrics and Gynecology at Brooklyn's Lutheran Medical Center, says, "There is a genetic component to labor and delivery ... but it is not always all that reliable. It's a very soft relationship. The place where there really is a true relationship is in medical complications in pregnancy, such as pre-eclampsia."

Dr. Hoskins says the shape of the pelvis, which partially determines how easy it will be for the baby to descend, is also genetically determined. But, of course, that means that a woman's father's DNA also plays a role. And then there are other factors, including the size of the baby, and its position in the pelvis, which can affect the speed and ease of delivery.

Not all surprises in childbirth are disappointments. Jodi had the kind of delivery most women dream about. "Oh my God, it was a piece of cake," she says of her quick, complication free-birth. David chimes in, "Ours was embarrassing. Even our doctor said, 'You might not want to tell people about this.'" Jodi adds, "I absolutely expected it to be excruciatingly painful and dramatic. Those birthing videos are pretty graphic and frightening. Plus, I've heard a lot of horror stories in the past – women who were in labor for 32 hours, emergency C-sections." She says it was easy compared with what she had been expecting. The hardest part of the day was figuring out whether or not she was in labor. Early that morning Jodi noticed, "I was peeing more often, and I called my husband and said, 'Is this it?' And he said, 'Well, I don't know.'"

When an expectant mother asks a woman who has already had children what labor feels like, the typical response is, "Oh, you'll know! You can't miss it!" Well, you can. We assume that a pregnant woman will know exactly when her body is ready to send a new life into the world. After all, how could she fail to notice something that is supposed to be so obvious? The problem is that the start of labor is not always apparent. Women are often prepared for some kind of alien experience, a foreign and powerful sensation, but sometimes those early contractions simply feel like a more intense version of regular menstrual cramps or a bad stomach virus. Some women's contractions are so slight they cannot even feel them. Since these sensations are not what they had been expecting, moms-to-be may overlook the beginning of labor.

The perception that labor is always evident can make some women feel foolish for failing to recognize that the momentous event they have been waiting for, dreaming about and stressing over has begun. But consider this: Sara, a young obstetrician practicing in New York City, a woman who has obviously spent years studying the female body and the reproductive processes, could not tell whether she herself was in labor. Women should take comfort knowing that sometimes the labor process confounds even the experts.

Cesarean sections

In 2003, the number of women who had cesarean sections in the United States increased by 5% to 27.5%, the highest rate ever recorded.[53] In England, about 23% of births are cesarean, with more than half qualifying as "emergency."[54] Shannon was 37 weeks pregnant when she had a cesarean section and says it was a bit of a let-down: "I felt like I didn't do what I was supposed to get to do. It wasn't a real birth. Like when people talk about giving birth, you feel like you didn't really give birth. But I did. The most important thing to me was the fact that the babies were fine," notes Shannon. She adds, "I kept just trying to tell myself, 'Things happen the way they were meant to be. This is what was meant to happen.'"

While some women view cesareans as a disappointment, and blame themselves for failing to achieve what they assume should be a completely natural act – a vaginal delivery – others consider a cesarean birth a blessing in disguise. Renee was thrilled to have one scheduled. She once nearly passed out after witnessing a vaginal birth while taking a nursing assistant course. "I just see myself as lucky," she says. "I mean no labor pains. How lucky can you get? I was just blessed. I was meant to have this baby this way."

Vanessa confesses that a cesarean section has benefits many women do not immediately consider. She recalls one of her friends talking about how painful her episiotomy was. "It took her a while for intercourse to start feeling good. It was actually still painful after a couple of months. ... Thank God [for the cesarean section]," laughs Vanessa.

Preemies

Parents of premature babies may feel as if the journey to parenthood has been abruptly cut short, that they did not get the time they had expected to prepare for their new responsibilities. Jessica, a 33-year-old mother who delivered her son at 28 weeks, says, "Mentally, you're not prepared for the pregnancy to be over."

About one in every eight babies born in the United States is premature, meaning the infant was born at less than 37 weeks of gestation.[55] Risk factors for premature delivery fall into a number of different categories. One category is a woman's obstetric history – whether she has had a previous premature birth, fertility problems, or become pregnant within less than six months of a previous delivery.[56] Chronic illness in the mother – such as diabetes, high blood pressure or kidney disease – as well as vaginal bleeding, malnutrition, a ruptured amniotic sac, obesity and being underweight before pregnancy can all increase the likelihood of a premature delivery. A woman who is pregnant with multiples has a greater chance of delivering early, as does an expectant mother with an incompetent cervix, fibroids, an abnormally shaped uterus or a baby with a major birth defect. Certain lifestyle behaviors are also linked with a higher risk, including smoking, drinking, using illegal drugs and not receiving proper prenatal care. However, nearly 50% of women who go into preterm labor have no known risk factors.[57]

Preterm birth is one of the leading causes of infant mortality in the United States.[58] Prematurity can lead to a number of short-term and long-term health problems, such as underdeveloped organs, respiratory difficulties, chronic lung disease, infections, mild to severe cerebral palsy, impaired hearing and vision, blindness and deafness. Yet, because of major advances in neonatal intensive care, doctors are now able to save babies who 15 years ago would not have survived.

Frequently, not only do parents of preemies have to deal with their babies' serious health problems, but they must also cope with having to leave their tiny infants behind in the hospital's neonatal intensive-care unit (NICU). The length of a NICU stay can range from a few days to months. The day she was discharged, Jessica was wheeling a cart of balloons and cards from well-wishers down to the lobby to meet her husband and leave the hospital. A woman who was escorting a joyful couple and their new baby out of the hospital looked at Jessica's cart and joked, "Oh, don't forget your baby!" Jessica burst into tears. "Obviously, more than anything, I wanted to take him home with me," says Jessica. "But as the parent of a preemie, you have to realize that there's no way you can possibly care for your child at home. There's nothing you can do about the situation. You just have to get through it. When you first leave the hospital, part of you is just so happy your child is alive."

Jennifer declares, "Being discharged without my babies was the worst day of my entire life. I was a nutcase. I thought my husband was going to have me committed." Her babies were born six weeks early via a cesarean section and spent 12 days in the hospital. "I felt like a bad mother because I was leaving them in the NICU." Jennifer says the NICU experience undermined her confidence as a mother and made her feel detached from her children. "I had to ask permission to hold my babies. I mean, I was treated like a visitor. You know what I mean? They did not treat me like I was their mother. My husband had a different experience. But I felt like I was basically being told what to do for them, not in a way that was teaching me, but in a way that was like, 'You don't know what you're doing.'" Jennifer's husband, Fred, appreciated the NICU's safe environment, where there were always trained professionals standing by to help. He explains, "We got good training on how to take care of them. We knew there was a lot of security there, that we couldn't really do anything wrong if the babies started crying or looked funny. There were nurses right there so you could ask, 'Is this right? Is there something wrong?' So taking them home was kind of like losing that security blanket."

Because preemies are born before their bodies have had time to develop fully, they are often dependent on machines to keep them alive, to help them breathe and eat, until their bodies mature. Some parents fear the NICU environment will hinder bonding. However, once a baby is strong enough, doctors will usually permit his parents to hold him. Many doctors and NICU nurses encourage what is known as "kangaroo care" – skin-to-skin contact, with the baby resting on the parent's chest or stomach. Kangaroo care was first introduced in Bogotá, Colombia, in the early 1980s and dramatically reduced the infant mortality rate there. Researchers say it leads to more rapid weight gain, shorter hospital stays and increased attachment between parent and baby.[59–61]

The baby's here! Reviewing the big debut

"Words don't do that feeling justice of seeing and then holding your firstborn child. ... It was as if I received the greatest gift a man could have," exclaims Ralph. For some newly anointed mothers and fathers, the birth is the be-all and end-all experience. "If, when I die, I can choose to go back to one time in my life, it would be the moment Elliot was born through to the next few hours," remarks Kate, continuing, "Everything just kind of fit into place. ... It was just the three of us, and the room was just really dark and still. Paul and I didn't really say anything to each other. We just sat there with him. And Paul took a couple of pictures of Elliot on me. ... It was my piece of heaven."

"When he finally came out, it was like watching a miracle," says New York dad Adrian of his son's birth. "It was completely emotional. I was ecstatic and crying and just amazed at what I was seeing. Definitely, looking back, it was one of the top moments of my life ... I was amazed, in awe. I couldn't believe that our baby was coming out."

For other parents, the moment of birth is anticlimactic, especially when they do not experience the emotional fireworks they had anticipated. "I remember imagining that there would be this burst of emotion and I'd be so overwhelmed because everybody we talked to had said, 'You're not going to believe the feeling when you see that baby,'" says Catherine. But, of her son Matthew's delivery, she notes, "I was in shock. ... There wasn't this big rush of tears, a *Hallmark*, *Oprah* kind of thing." Catherine, who produces television commercials and music videos, talked about her baby's birth as if it were one of her projects: "It was like, 'OK, cut. It's a wrap. We're done. Let's just clean up. The production is over.'"

Sometimes a parent may be disappointed about the baby's gender. Single mom Renee says, "I wanted a girl. I wanted a buddy. When I found out it was a boy, I thought, 'What am I going to do with a boy? I'm a single mother. What am I going to do with a boy? How am I going to potty train him? What am I going to do about sports? I don't know shit about sports.'" But she concedes, "God has a plan and a reason for everything. Everybody keeps telling me that it's going to be cheaper for me financially in the long-run. They also say boys love their mothers."

A parent also may be less than impressed with her infant's initial appearance. Keri says little Cooper "looked like a miniature sumo wrestler. He was just so fat. I didn't think he was that cute, which I can't believe I'm saying with him now being in the same room. Poor guy! But once we got home, he lost a few pounds right away. Then he started looking like a normal little baby."

Wande echoes Keri's sentiments: "I guess I was more in shock than anything. I thought, 'Wow! This baby *isn't* really cute.' But none of them are when they come out. They all look extraterrestrial. But you see the parenting magazines and all the newborns look alike. They don't really depict what a one-minute-old baby looks like." They don't look "all wrinkly and weird looking," as Wande puts it. There is a good reason. The "newborn" babies we see in magazines, as well as in movies and on television shows, are typically not newborns.

"Usually, the 'newborn' babies we use are anywhere from 3 months to 5 months old," explains Chris O'Shea, a baby wrangler and stylist for magazines and print advertisements. As a baby wrangler, it is her job to make sure that the babies on the set of a photo or television commercial shoot are content, so the photographer can get a good shot. "When photographing babies, we need them to have some sort of response and reaction. ... And before the age of 3 months, because everything is so primary for them, they just can't respond in the way that we need them to, with the smiles and reactions and expressions that we really need for photographs," says O'Shea, who has worked for almost every major parenting magazine in the United States, as well as some of the biggest names in children's retail and baby-care products.

Many parents would argue that even if a newborn is not ready for a casting call, he is still picture-perfect material. Kate says, "Elliot had a cone head because he had a ventouse. He had curly black hair stuck to the top of his head. It was hilarious. It was just kind of glued to his head. And he had really, really red lips. He sounds really gross, but he was absolutely stunning." Her husband, Paul, recalls, "I had been quite stressed because I knew that I had to tell Katy what the sex of the baby was. So that was the first thing on my mind." But it was not the first thing on little Elliot's mind. Paul says, "I saw him come out and put my hand on his bum for some reason. I don't know why [I did that]. And then he [went to the bathroom] in my hand. So my first reaction was, 'Thanks very much. That was lovely.'"

CHAPTER 6

Welcoming baby

When Kate and Paul brought Elliot home from the hospital, they sat down in their living room, placed Elliot, still strapped in his car-seat carrier, between them and just stared at him. "We just kind of sat there and said 'What do we do now?'" recalls Kate. David and Jodi had an almost identical conversation 5,400 miles away in Los Angeles. David remembers, "The first day that Tess came home, we were sitting here, the three of us, and we were in her bedroom and we said, 'What the hell do we do now? She's awake and we're sitting here and what in God's name do we do now?'"

New parents can feel as if they are stuck in a surreal fog. They may wonder, "How can we *not* know what to do after nine months of exhaustive preparation?" They attended baby-care classes, read all the latest parenting books, scanned countless parenting websites and listened to seemingly endless advice (much of it unsolicited) from practically everyone they encountered during the pregnancy. And yet they are at a loss. Should they feed the baby? Entertain him? Cuddle him? Do they need to "do anything" with him, or is he fine just lying there, taking in the sights and sounds of his new home? Jodi recollects her terror the first day home from the hospital. David had an audition so she was left to fend for herself. He was gone for only an hour, but Jodi says that it felt like an eternity. "I'm in the bedroom with Tess, and I'm beside myself. I'm so nervous, I'm so scared. I don't know what to do. So I just sat in the room with the baby until my husband came home."

The sometimes overwhelming initiation into parenthood can make first-time parents feel as if their little bundle of joy is running his own "shock and awe" campaign from the bassinet perched in the middle of the living room. Never could they have imagined how one tiny little person would cause such unimaginable chaos. LeeRan confesses, "I thought it was going to be really easy. He'd eat and sleep, and then I'd sleep. I did not think it was going to be that hard." However, their infant Matthew had other ideas about his schedule, none of which included much sleeping. "That first night I was up every hour and thought, 'Oh my God. What did I do?'" says LeeRan. Her husband, Tim, remarks, "You can't prepare yourself for the changes. It's been a shock. It's been a good shock, but it's been unreal."

Caring for the newest family member

Stacey says that after she and Loren brought Lainey home from the hospital,

"We were scared to death that we were going to break her neck." Loren adds, "I did not feel capable of keeping her alive." The next morning they breathed a collective sigh of relief upon seeing that Lainey had indeed survived the night. Dino also worried about accidentally harming his tiny baby girl: "She was so small. I was afraid I was going to hurt her by handling her too roughly. Just feeding her was intense because I had this fear of hurting her."

Fears of dropping, breaking and hurting the baby are all typical. Even Leslie, a medical doctor, was nervous about caring for her newborn son. She says, "The practical things like how to give him a bath and how to clean him up properly after a dirty diaper, those things freaked me out. I've got four years of medical education, but they don't teach you how to do the everyday stuff." Leslie also talks about another typical fear of new parents – cutting the baby's fingernails without slicing off a finger. "I was terrified of cutting his nails. I put it off for three weeks. I couldn't do it. That little nail clipper is the scariest tool. I wait until he's asleep. Even then I can only do like two nails. But he hasn't scratched himself up too bad so I must be doing something right," she jokes.

Dr. Palmo Pasquariello, a pediatrician with Global Pediatrics in New York City, has been practicing for 18 years and has seen about 20,000 newborns. Asked what new parents' typical concerns are, he replied, "They want to make sure the baby's breathing, the baby's not breathing too fast, the baby's eating enough, the baby's not sick, the baby's not sleeping too much, [or] too little. Basically it's an entirely new organism, and they have no idea what baseline is until they get to know their kid for a while. So we try to give them some parameters." He says parents want to know when to worry and when to relax. "We try to give them basic guidelines in terms of temperatures and respiratory rates and amounts of wet diapers and amounts of ounces the babies need to eat, without trying to overwhelm them with information."

Although sudden infant death syndrome, or SIDS, is rare, affecting fewer than 1 in 1,000 babies born each year, it is frequently the number-one fear of new parents.[62] It is common for a new parent to find herself periodically racing to the nursery to check whether her infant is still breathing. Sometimes it is hard to tell just by looking at a newborn, since infants can be very quiet, shallow breathers. So parents will devise their own special tests. Dr. Pasquariello explains, "They put a little Q-tip under the nose to see if the cotton moves, or they see if the make-up mirror fogs up." Researchers are still at a loss to explain the exact cause of SIDS. But the rate of SIDS has declined by 50% since 1992, when the American Academy of Pediatrics started recommending that parents put their babies to sleep on their backs, rather than on their sides or stomachs.[63]

Breastfeeding

Breastfeeding can also be a source of considerable stress for women. Catherine assumed she would have no trouble. She believed breastfeeding was such a natural and straightforward process that any woman could easily master it. Then she tried it. "Breastfeeding has been challenging," she admits. "You think, 'How hard could it be?' ... The baby's got a mouth, you've got a breast. He'll latch right on there. The most challenging thing is dealing with the soreness, the actual physical damage. My right side, just dealing with the cracking, it's so painful and frustrating." Initially discouraged, Catherine says, "I started to feel like, 'Maybe I can't do this.' And yet I felt that if I were to go to formula, I'd feel like a failure." She was convinced she could make it work, and sought the assistance of La Leche League International, a worldwide organization offering breastfeeding "peer counseling" from other mothers. Catherine's determination eventually paid off, and she can now share what she calls that "special moment" with her son without all of the discomfort. She says that if she had given up on breastfeeding, she would have felt that she had somehow compromised her baby's health by depriving him of nutrient-rich breast milk.

With all of the pressure today to breastfeed, women who are unable to, or who do not want to, sometimes feel as if they have failed their babies. The myths surrounding breastfeeding include: Every woman can and should breastfeed. Good mothers breastfeed. And, breastfeeding is essential for bonding. Researchers at the University of Kent, England, interviewed 500 women about their attitudes on breastfeeding. Sixty-three percent of the women agreed with the statement "If a woman can successfully breastfeed, then she should do so."[64] The truth is that although the American Academy of Pediatrics endorses at least a full year of breastfeeding, it may not be right for everyone. (A survey conducted by the Centers for Disease Control and Prevention (CDC) found that only 39% of babies were still breastfed at 6 months of age.)[65] What a baby needs most from his mother is love, affection and a sense of security. A mother who has no physical problems that preclude her from breastfeeding may choose not to because she does not want her husband to feel left out, she believes breastfeeding desexualizes the breasts, or she fears that her husband will no longer see her as a sexual individual. Additionally, a woman may not want to breastfeed because she is embarrassed, or has concerns about time constraints and complications once she returns to work.

Mark supported Catherine in her efforts to nurse but felt excluded when she was breastfeeding exclusively. Things changed once Catherine started pumping, and he could give Matthew a bottle. "To have that connection with him and have him stare at me while I'm feeding him, it's fantastic. You look at him, he's staring at you. You feel in your heart that he's feeling so safe and he's feeling so good right now because he's eating, and you're the one who's feeding him," Mark exclaims. A new dad who is concerned about being sidelined because of breastfeeding should be aware that his encouragement can increase his partner's chances of successfully breastfeeding. His reassurance can help his wife (or partner) relax, and that facilitates milk production.

The learning curve: maintaining perspective

Ensuring the survival of another human being is an awesome responsibility, but one that is infinitely more manageable than many new parents assume it will be. Six weeks postpartum, LeeRan says, "It's so much better. I'm just used to being up. I know that I will have to get up. I know how to set him back down to sleep. And I can tell if he's hungry when he's crying or if he's just tired. ... I have my little tricks now that I feel like I know him a little more."

Five weeks after giving birth to Matthew, Catherine notes, "You develop your language with each other. You learn what they want and how to respond. You have to find your rhythm as a mother, as a baby, as a couple and as a family. All these things have to click." The "language" that Catherine speaks of is called *attunement*. It is the mother's growing capacity to assess what her baby needs and then to react accordingly.

Kate and Paul conquered the new parenting learning curve by devising their own special strategy. "Paul and I just said, 'Everything we do for the first time, we'll do together. The first nappies, we'll do together. The first bath, we'll do together.' Paul was off work for about three weeks when Elliot came home, so we just kind of worked through everything together," explains Kate. Paul admits that he had never been much of a "baby person" until Elliot arrived. "I'd never held a baby before in my life. I never ever dreamed of holding a baby because they just scared me rigid. I was always scared that I'd drop them or hurt them or squeeze them too tight. I wouldn't even hold my god-daughter. And I don't know what changed with Elliot. It's almost as if I knew that I just had to do it." And so Paul had no qualms about holding his own son. "It's like having a really expensive china pot," he says. "If it's yours, you don't mind picking it up. But if it's someone else's, then you're worried about dropping it."

Paul acknowledges that while Elliot was still in the hospital, he was nervous about caring for him in front of the trained professionals. "The midwife said, 'Do you want to help change his nappy? Do you want to help wash him?' And I said, 'No, no, no. I'm fine. I'll just watch you. I need to learn how to do it.' But that was basically my way of saying, 'I'm a bit embarrassed because I've never done it before, and I don't want to make an idiot of myself.' But once we got him home and it was just me and Katy, there was no embarrassment. You're both in the same boat, so you just get on with it."

Many new parents experience feelings of anxiety and helplessness when they cannot figure out just why their babies are acting a certain way – crying incessantly, not sleeping or eating. They feel powerless to make things right when they cannot even determine what is wrong. And there is nothing more frustrating than trying to control the uncontrollable. As Kelly says, "It's all been traumatic. Roberto freaks out, too. We freak out when she's crying or when she's having gas pains. That's been really hard, the colic and not knowing what is wrong with her. And Roberto freaks out, says we're horrible parents and we don't know what we're doing. We've been to the pediatrician twice because of the colic, and Roberto wants a solution and there is no solution. We're learning – which I already knew – that there are a lot of gray areas, not black and white. He's having a harder time, wanting a black-and-white solution, and it just doesn't exist." Roberto says he would not describe the experience as traumatic but admits, "I freaked out. ... We love Emma but we felt like, 'Is she possessed?' because she was crying and it didn't seem normal. She was wailing." Kelly breaks in, laughing, "Yeah, we called her the devil child. Roberto was like, 'Should we call the priest?'" "Nobody tells you that this is normal," says Roberto. "Then you go to the pediatrician, you talk to other people and you find out that the first few months, it's like that. So, OK, she's normal. There's nothing wrong with her."

Some parents experience performance anxiety when it comes time to care for their newborns. They forget everything they have read and learned about babies. It is as if they have lost the instructions to some expensive new gadget they have just purchased and are afraid to explore on their own, worried that they will cause irreparable damage. First-time parents will eventually find out that a new baby is a lot more resilient than he looks. Every new parent will have at least one heart-stopping moment when the baby accidentally topples off the couch, or rolls from the changing table onto the floor. New parents should rest assured because these incidents are usually far more traumatic for them than for their babies.

It is no mystery that new parents have trouble maintaining a sense of perspective amidst the chaotic postpartum period. But the turmoil does ultimately end. In time, the baby will sleep through the night, and a new parent will recognize which of the baby's cues signal that he is tired, hungry or gassy. As parents become better at reading their infants, more competent at diapering, feeding, soothing and bathing their babies, they will gain confidence in their parenting abilities. Sooner or later, the new family unit will establish some kind of routine, thereby adding the comfort and predictability that most of us – even babies – need and crave. Things do eventually fall into place, whether it takes six weeks or six months. There is no hard and fast deadline.

The only thing that is predictable about parenthood is that it is unpredictable. An infant who sleeps almost non-stop during his first two weeks home from the hospital, will not necessarily turn out to be a good sleeper. (A baby's sleep patterns can change every few weeks.) A baby who refuses a bottle for the first few months may later be so attached to it that he has a hard time giving it up before his second birthday. Often the transition to parenthood is a smoother one if a new mother or father is able to see past these temporary frustrations and focus on the bigger picture. It can become especially important to adopt such a long-term outlook when a new parent is coping with additional life stresses, such as a death in the family, a divorce or other hardship.

Kemba and Camara delivered their baby at 3:03 am on August 30, 2005 in New Orleans, a day shy of 28 weeks. This was less than 24 hours after

Hurricane Katrina, the biggest natural disaster to hit the United States in more than a century, pummeled the city.

Kemba delivered her little boy in the interior section of the hospital, the only area that still had power, thanks to a generator. Kemba says it was so hot and uncomfortable that people began breaking windows to let in the fresh air. "On top of that, you didn't know what was going to happen. ... It's like, 'OK, your baby's there on life support. If the hospital runs out of generator power, what happens to him?'"

Luckily, Kemba never had to find out. Fifteen hours after he was born, 2.2-pound Camara Jr. ("C.J.") and the ventilator he needed in order to breathe were airlifted to the Woman's Hospital in Baton Rouge, Louisiana. His parents could not go with him. Kemba was evacuated the next day by boat and was extremely relieved to be reunited with C.J. in Baton Rouge that afternoon. But she did not see her husband or mother, a dialysis patient, until three days later. Because Kemba was a hospital patient, she was evacuated first, without them. Kemba's mother and Camara were evacuated later the same day by two men with a fan boat. Their rescuers dropped them off on a dry street corner, leaving them to find their own way out of the devastated city. The two hiked about three miles to the convention center. Camara describes the scene: "There were people all over the place who had no idea where to go. They were hauling people in like herds of cattle into the backs of trucks and just dropping them off at the convention center. And it was very chaotic. People had no sense of direction, no sense of where to go. They were basically telling us to stay there, and buses were going to come, but the buses never came."

The two spent one night at the convention center before making their way to a relative's house in New Orleans. Kemba says none of their cell phones were working. The three of them were able to make only out-of-state calls from the landlines. So her husband and mother would phone a cousin in Dallas, who would then conference in Kemba in Baton Rouge. That was their only means of communication, and the only way for Kemba to update her husband on the status of their premature son. "You didn't have time to sit and think what was going to happen next. All you could do was kind of take a breath and keep going," notes Kemba.

Three days after leaving the New Orleans hospital, a helicopter transported Camara and his mother-in-law to the airport, where members of their church picked them up and drove them to Baton Rouge so that Camara could join his wife and C.J. Of her reaction upon seeing her husband, Kemba says, "I don't even know if I can put that into words. ... Actually, seeing that he was fine and he was OK. ... It was unexplainable." She says for him to be able to see his son fighting for his life was an incredible feeling.

Kemba advises other new parents going through a hardship to "account for what's important, and the rest will take care of itself." She adds, "Being a new mom is great. We don't take any moment for granted. We try to enjoy our time with him as much as we possibly can because it's really only the grace of God that allowed him to be here, allowed him to be in good health. And he's doing so well."

Bonding

"I felt like as soon as she was on my chest, it was like, 'OK, that's it. I'm a mom. She's my daughter. Here we go,'" says Stacey of her instant bond with Lainey. David says it took him "seven seconds" to bond with his daughter, Tess. Bonding can be immediate, or it may take a few weeks. The bonding between parent and baby is the development of an intense, powerful, emotional connection. A parent experiences an overwhelming desire to protect her baby and envelop him with love and affection. New parents should not feel guilty if this bond is not instantaneous and automatic, as we are so often led to believe it should be. It can take time to get to know a baby and to form a relationship with him or her. Although there is no precise schedule, a mother who continues to feel disconnected and detached beyond two weeks might want to discuss her feelings with someone she trusts, such as a family member or close friend, her obstetrician or a therapist. Sometimes emotional detachment is a symptom of postpartum depression.

For Leslie, the chaos of the first few weeks postpartum put a damper on bonding. "I was just so scared. I was scared I was going to break him every time I touched him. I was scared he wasn't eating enough. I was scared the breastfeeding wasn't going as well as I wanted it to. I spent so much time being scared that I think bonding was the last thing on my mind. It was just like, 'Let me get through the first few weeks,'" she comments. "The baby nurse sort of taught me the ropes. I felt more of the attachment stuff once the fear subsided a little bit, and now it's growing every day." Leslie says that at first she felt guilty after she did not achieve an instantaneous bond. "I felt kind of selfish for being so sidetracked by my fears about everything. I thought, 'God, I should have thought about this already. I should have come to terms with this already. I should have thought about this before he was born.'"

Marla, a Laguna beach, California mom, also acknowledges that after Jacob was born, "I didn't feel the connection right away. But breastfeeding really helped me to connect to him because that was our alone time together. ... No one bothered us, especially during the night feedings. There were no other sounds or people, and we could really focus on each other during that time. I really started to get to know him and talk to him and dream about what he was going to do when he grows up ... I still feel like we have a special connection because of that alone time," she says two years after Jacob's birth.

D.J. says that it took a boys' "bachelor" weekend before he felt a true bond with Cooper. He explains, "It's really the weirdest thing. Watching him be born, and then watching them put Cooper in Keri's arms with the cord still attached, I was just a mess. But I don't think I connected to his personality – if that makes any sense – until he was probably two months old. I was connected to him as a baby, and I was crying my eyes out when Keri was holding him. But as far as connecting to him as a person, it was probably when she went on her first business trip. For two days, I did everything with him. That's when daddy and son really hit it off. We watched a Reds game every single night she was gone. I think I enjoyed it more than he did, but it was good. ... Now when she leaves, it's like old home week. And he and I, we 'bach' it. That's what we call it when she's gone – we're bachelors."

There are a number of different ways a father can begin to connect with his baby during the early weeks. He can cradle her, read or sing to her, and bathe her. He can also feed her if his partner is not solely breastfeeding. Men need not feel left out of the bonding equation just because they cannot breastfeed.

New division of labor: who's doing what

Nearly every new parent will admit that having a baby involves a tremendous amount of work. The baby has to be fed, burped and changed every few hours. These tasks create a whole slew of secondary chores – bottles need to be sterilized and washed, breast milk pumped, dirty diapers disposed of, sheets and clothes constantly washed. And then there are still the basic household responsibilities that need to be handled. Someone must pay the bills, buy groceries, cook, send in the dry cleaning, and clean the house. It seems as if a new parent can never check off every item on the "to-do" list.

The key to tackling the never-ending list of chores is to divide and conquer, which is exactly what Leslie and Peter did during the early weeks postpartum. Leslie notes, "We put Peter in charge of the food. Peter did all of the food shopping. Whenever he didn't cook, we would order in, which we did a lot. I think we could've kept all the neighborhood restaurants in business ourselves!" Leslie's mother took laundry duty and ran errands.

Scott Coltrane, a sociology professor at the University of California, Riverside, focuses on family and gender issues. He says that when it comes to caring for a newborn, "Oftentimes, the mother's identity is tied up with learning – particularly with a first child – learning how to be a good mother, wanting enough interaction time, wanting to be the expert at doing whatever it is with the child. And sometimes men allow the women to have special bonds with the kids and begin to remove themselves a little bit. And so it takes a lot of effort on the man's part to stay involved after the birth." He offers an example of when the baby is crying in the middle of the night. "So why not have a division of labor where the father is the one who always gets up and gets the baby and brings it to the mother if she's breastfeeding? There are little things that couples can do, but it takes some assertion on the part of the father usually, but also facilitation on the part of the mother. She has to plan for his inclusion." This limitation on the father's involvement is called "maternal gatekeeping," which is defined in a study by researchers at Brigham Young University as "a collection of beliefs and behaviors that ultimately inhibit a collaborative effort between men and women in family work by limiting men's opportunities [to participate in housework and childcare]."[66]

Although men today are more involved in baby care than their own fathers were, it is still typically the mother who takes time off from work to care for the new baby. Maternity leave can be particularly stressful and isolating for a woman who is accustomed to working outside the home. At first, Leslie, a doctor, and LeeRan, a high-level planning promoter at a Fortune 500 company, each felt that they were struggling alone with new motherhood. They were home on maternity leave while their husbands went off to work each day, continuing their pre-baby lives. Leslie had decided to take a year off before starting a residency in emergency medicine. She recalls feeling a little jealous when Peter was getting ready for work one day shortly after the baby was born. She recounts: "One morning he was putting on his tie, and he was halfway out the door and he said, 'I love you guys, I'll see you later,' and I just started crying. He said, 'What's the matter?' And I said, 'Look at you. You get to go.' And I was still in pain at that point and a lot of other confounding factors. And I'm now at the point where it's not a negative thing. I'm just envious that he doesn't have to pump, and that he doesn't have to think about what to do all day."

Six weeks postpartum, LeeRan complains that while her husband's life hasn't changed much, her world has been turned upside down. "I don't think he quite gets what I'm doing, what I get done around the house, that he gets to leave and I don't get to leave." LeeRan says Tim has more freedom and more control over his own time. Her schedule is dictated by that of the baby. She was particularly upset about a weekend golf outing Tim took with his buddies, and how he managed to leave work early for the trip. "It is funny to me," notes LeeRan with a hint of sarcasm, "he can get home early for things like that, but can't get home early on a regular basis to help with the baby and house-work." Tim responds, "I probably take things for granted with her. ... We men are kind of dumb. We don't know how to read women." He continues, "My life for all intents and purposes, from the time I go to work in the morning until the time I go home, has been unchanged. However, it has changed when I get home at night. I can't just lie on the couch and watch a ball game."

Visitors: the fan club

New parents are not the only ones who want to welcome the baby into the world. Typically, friends, family members, colleagues and mere acquaintances all want to share in what is billed as the ultimate blessed and joyous occasion: the birth of a new baby.

Consequently, a couple may feel as if they are running a bed-and-breakfast, catering to streams of well-wishers that flow to and from their home. Handling all the guests, especially the overnight ones, is yet another "job" for over-burdened new parents. Kelly says it is very helpful having her mother-in-law stay with them. But she questions whether the disadvantages outweigh the advantages. "I love her. I think she's a great woman. She's very sweet, very nurturing – she lives for her children. But I've had to deal with some criticism and some things that were probably said behind my back." Asked if this chipped away at her sense of security as a mother, Kelly laughingly responded, "No, it just makes me want her to leave." Roberto has a very different perspective on the situation. He says to Kelly, "My mother told me the other day 'I feel like a stranger in my own son's house.' But she's trying. She only appears if you call her. She only participates if you let her. She tries not to make any noise. She tries to cook anytime she can. And I don't think you've been very appreciative of what she's done. Imagine how the house would look." Kelly interrupts, "That's what they care about, how the house would look." Roberto continues, "But really, imagine how the house would be and what we would be eating if she wasn't here and I'm going to work." In response, Kelly says, "The problem is she's not my priority." It is hard to make guests a priority when one is caring for a demanding newborn and has little or no time to care for oneself.

One of the mothers interviewed requested that her name not be used in this section to avoid upsetting her parents. This woman's mother came to stay with her and her husband in their two-bedroom apartment the second night after they brought the baby home from the hospital. The new mother confesses, "I felt like I had to cater to my parents, make sure that they were happy and getting enough time with my baby. And yet I was emotional that first week. It was not good. I just felt like I had to worry about what everybody else was thinking and feeling, and, meanwhile, all I wanted to do was focus on myself, my husband and my new baby. It was a little stressful."

Jim and Janine hosted their mothers, at different times, in their New York City apartment. "They weren't much help at all," comments Janine. "My mom is not familiar with New York City, she's very overweight and has emphysema, so it was hard for her to walk around and get groceries or do that type of thing." Janine says that because it is in her nature to want to make everyone feel comfortable, she cooked for her mother and mother-in-law and ran errands for them. Jim notes that his mother had a very hands-off attitude when it came to helping with the baby. "Like, 'Oh, I've changed enough diapers in my life. You've got to learn some time.' She was there physically, but by and large she was not a big help as far as the things we needed her to do. ... She was just there to spend time and watch the child, or to look at it, not to really give us a break. Maybe those were just my own expectations, or maybe I should have been clearer about what we needed help with. I thought it would've been apparent, but I guess not," says Jim.

Feeling pressure to play host is one problem new parents may have when people come to visit their baby. Others are that guests bring germs into the house, prevent parents from resting, and interfere with the parent-baby bonding process. Plus, everyone wants a chance to hold the baby. D.J. was particularly concerned about the "new baby hand-off." "If we gave Cooper to a relative, I was the one who freaked out about his head being held up. I'm the person who would say to family members, 'Watch his head, watch his head,' knowing they have 18 kids of their own. And they would say, 'I know, I got the hint.'"

The peanut gallery: the last word on advice

A new parent can get caught in an advice quandary. She (or he) may desperately want to ask others for tips on baby care, but is afraid that asking implies incompetence. However, there is nothing wrong with seeking advice from those who may have valuable wisdom to impart. It can be comforting to hear that one is not the only parent in the world who is unable to get her baby to nap for more than 20 minutes at a time.

Rookie parents should be prepared for an onslaught of advice. First-time mothers and fathers are magnets for it, particularly the unsolicited, unwanted kind. There is just something about an infant and her seemingly helpless parents that compels people to offer their two cents. Grandparents, in-laws, friends and co-workers who are already parents, single friends who have extensive babysitting experience, even strangers on the street, all feel the need to counsel new parents on the *right* way to care for a newborn. These "advisors" readily provide tips on breastfeeding (some never having breastfed a baby), getting the baby to sleep, and soothing and stimulating him. They also attempt to "educate" the newly initiated parent about the fine arts of diapering, burping and swaddling. Although these advice givers usually have good intentions, they do not realize that their suggestions can erode a new parent's confidence. In addition, these impromptu consultants are forgetting three crucial facts: every baby is different; no one knows a child better than his own parents; and there is often more than one way to achieve the same result.

Not wanting to hear anyone's words of wisdom, Wande refused the help of friends and family members after she and Dino first brought England home from the hospital. "I didn't feel like hearing everybody's ideas on how I should care for my child." But she could not isolate herself completely. "I did hear it. I just didn't hear it that soon. It just makes you feel inadequate, like you don't know what you're doing, or you don't know how to raise your own child. I know they didn't mean any harm by it, but I'm the type of person who takes it personally. I just want to snap at people."

Loren remembers people bombarding him with suggestions shortly after Lainey was born. It was practically parenting by committee, with each issue worthy of a G8 Summit. Loren lists some of the subjects that were up for debate: "the layers of clothes that should be on the child, whether the child should be wearing socks to bed or not, whether I should have a clean-shaven face so I wouldn't scratch the baby." Although they were grateful for their parents' help, Loren and Stacey say it is difficult to parent when one's own parents still want to be in charge. Loren explains: "Everyone meant well, but we had just become parents and wanted to be empowered and feel confident. I think it totally takes the air out of your tires, diminishes your confidence, when you're being told by your parents their thoughts. Part of it also was that you just want to say, 'Look, you had your time to be a parent. That was for us. Now it's our time. Let us enjoy it. Let us work through it, experience everything there is to experience without being told what to do or how to feel.'"

One of the most common pieces of advice first-time parents are likely to hear is: "Sleep when the baby sleeps." It sounds like a good theory, until a parent is faced with a baby who does not tend to sleep in large chunks of time. Some babies doze off for just 20 minutes, and a catnap is practically worthless to a new parent who may want to use those precious 1,200 seconds to shower, go to the bathroom or eat a meal. Shannon, mother of twins Nate and Owen, recalls, "People would say to me, 'Why don't you just nap when the babies nap?' And I thought, 'Well, when do the *babies* nap? What do you mean?'" The people giving Shannon advice were usually parents with only one child. "And I would think, 'Yeah, you have no idea. They never sleep at the same time.'"

A postpartum game plan

Expectant parents can spare themselves some of the postpartum chaos by planning ahead. Pregnancy is the time to mobilize one's resources. Recruit a friend or relative, or hire a baby nurse, doula and/or housekeeper to assist with the tremendous workload in the early postpartum period. Most expectant couples assume that they will need help for only the first week or two before they can manage on their own. But arranging for consistent help for the first four to six weeks will give new parents much-needed time to adjust and ease into this life-changing transition. Although any help is a significant benefit to new parents, sometimes delegating chores to a relative or friend is much more difficult than asking a paid employee to handle these tasks. With overnight guests, it is crucial to clarify expectations ahead of time and to find out how long they will be staying, what they will be doing, and what they will not be doing.

After the baby comes home, a new mother needs to be mothered, to be taken care of so that she can heal and have energy to care for her newborn. She should even pamper herself – dash out for a quick manicure or facial, or simply unwind in a nice long bath. The couple might want to find a relative or friend to babysit so that they can go out on a date and reconnect with each other.

New parents should not forget to take care of themselves. That means cutting themselves some slack when they do not accomplish all that they expect during a harried, exhausting day with their newborn. Leslie says, "At the end of the day, even if I haven't checked more than one thing off my 20-item-long to-do list, I remind myself – and I really feel it's true – that I have accomplished something because he's happy, he's healthy, he's dry, and he doesn't have anything wrong with him."

CHAPTER 7

The changing marital relationship

"When we celebrated our third anniversary, Nathan was almost 3 months old. And for our anniversary, Jim gave me a card that had a baby's butt on it, which was just an adorable, cute card. But, right away, I saw that and I thought, 'Oh my gosh! I'm not his wife anymore. I'm the mother of his child,'" reflects Janine. She continues, "And from what I understand, he didn't even really think about it. He just saw this really cute card. ... But then when I saw it, I thought, 'I'm not your lover anymore or your wife. I'm this mom.'"

Jim chimes in, "I was standing at the *Hallmark* store. I had looked through every other stupid card, and the one I ended up with was one I just happened to spot that touched my heart as I was walking out of the store empty-handed. It was just kind of weird the way it happened, how she interpreted it and how I gravitated toward it. There definitely was a period of time where instantaneously she went from being my lover to Nathan's mom, and slowly we're gravitating toward a balance there. It was definitely a struggle for both of us."

Jim and Janine both emphasize that they began their journeys to parenthood with a solid, marital foundation and were always very open with each other. Yet the stresses and strains of caring for a new baby were considerable enough to rattle even that strong foundation. Janine says, "We bickered. We said these crazy things to each other that we never did before. And, of course, when you're nagging someone or having that kind of challenge go on, and that additional stress, it's not foreplay by any means. You know what I mean?"

It is no wonder that there is often a decline in marital satisfaction following the birth of a couple's first child.[67–69] New parents tend to be exhausted and anxious as they adjust to parenthood and all the additional responsibilities that come with it. Leslie, mother of 7-week-old William, says, "I really have to make an effort to remember the big picture in our lives and what we want it to look like. It's so easy to get caught up in details. I feel like that was never a problem before. It was never this hard to maintain perspective. But now it can seem like the worst thing in the world if Peter doesn't empty the bag of dirty diapers. I'll think, 'Why am I always the one to empty the diaper bag? This is horrible.'" She continues, "But then I'll say to myself, 'Take a deep breath. Back up. Peter was just out of town for two days. It's okay that he didn't empty the diaper bag because he took out the garbage, he emptied the dishwasher and he made dinner. So don't forget all of that good stuff just because there's one little thing that's annoying you.' So that's really a challenge now like it never was before."

Jay Belsky, an internationally-recognized scholar in the field of family research, is the Director of the Institute for the Study of Children, Families and Social Issues at Birkbeck College, University of London. He emphasizes that couples need to appreciate "how important and central and never-ending" the issues surrounding the division of labor will be. "The thing about the division of labor is it's relentless. It doesn't go away. It's there every morning, every afternoon, every evening. If one partner isn't satisfied with their sexual intimacy, or the frequency of it, or the quality of it, that's not something that's there all the time. It may be there when you climb into bed a couple of times a week, but the laundry, the diaper changing, the food shopping, the cleaning, those are there all the time. They don't go away. So it's almost like metaphorically, but right on target, there's always a toy to trip over," Belsky says.

A newborn can alter the household division of labor from whatever comfortable arrangement was in place before she came along. Her arrival means her parents are in for an incredible amount of work. It is all hands on deck, even if all those hands are not used to being on deck. Redefining roles and determining who does what can be particularly stressful, especially when a new mother and father have not shared their expectations with each other. Who is in charge of night-time feedings? Who is responsible for grocery shopping? Who will re-stock the diaper drawer?

Today couples have more choices about how to organize their lives once they have children. "Couples have to negotiate a lot more," says Professor Coltrane. "[The division of labor] is not all set. We're not inheriting. It's not just the way your mother did it or the way your grandmother did it. You have to talk about it, and that's hard on relationships." He adds, "It's hard on men, who generally have less practice being open emotionally. And there are special stresses on women because they're generally considered to be the ones who are responsible for maintaining harmony in the relationship. They don't want to be fighting all the time. So they have to evaluate: 'Should I ask him to do this one thing? He's not volunteering to do it. Should I offer to do it for him? Should I just do it for him without talking about it? Should I raise it as one of the negotiated issues?'"

Researchers once described the transition to parenthood as a crisis.[70–72] Even though the act of creating a new life together can cement an emotional bond between parents, the months surrounding childbirth can be one of the most stressful times in a couple's relationship. Roles change, physical and emotional demands increase, and the focus shifts from each other to the baby. A couple's need for physical intimacy, as well as their previously established patterns of relating to each other, are inevitably affected. Moreover, any major life change, even the ones that bring us extreme pleasure, implies some type of loss – a loss of what was, a loss of life as it previously existed. A new baby means a loss of time – couple time, personal time, work time, time spent with friends – as well as a loss of freedom and familiar routine.

Competing loyalties

"I used to be the screensaver on Dino's computer, and now it's our daughter who's the screensaver," jests a good-humored Wande. To borrow the tag line from Johnson & Johnson's baby-care commercials, "Having a baby changes everything." Once the baby arrives, it is easy to feel like the odd man – or woman – out. When a couple transforms their two-person unit into a three-person family, loyalties may shift. The partner may not be the one who automatically comes first anymore. And that can be hard to handle.

For many women, the birth of a first child is the most profound of all emotional experiences. They have never before experienced such a capacity to love and sacrifice. The renowned British pediatrician and psychoanalyst D.W. Winnicott wrote that in the last part of a woman's pregnancy and the early postnatal weeks she will experience "primary maternal preoccupation" as she essentially withdraws from the world in a "fugue"-like state. During this period of "heightened sensitivity," she focuses on the needs of her newborn.[73]

Primary maternal preoccupation is only a temporary state. But the birth of a baby can lead to a more permanent shift in family priorities. Wande admits, "I think once you have kids, your whole focus is different. My allegiance is first to my daughter." Of her two roles, Wande says, "I'm a mom first and a wife second." As Wande explains her reasons for putting her daughter first, she alludes to a news story she heard about the plight of an Australian mother who was vacationing with her family in Thailand when the devastating tsunami hit in December 2004. Wande says that when the wall of water washed over the resort island of Phuket, "There was a mother who was holding both of her kids, and she had to make the decision to let go of one to save two lives, instead of all three of them perishing. So she had to let go of one of her kids." Wande thinks about what she would do if she were ever in a similar situation, only she had to choose between saving her husband or saving her daughter. "I keep saying to myself, 'Lord forgive me if I were ever in the same situation.' I couldn't let my child die before an adult. So I would have to let go of my husband, as much as I love him. Blood is blood. But I would want him to make the same decision if he were ever in that position. I would want him to make sure England was taken care of." (Incidentally, the little boy the Australian mother let go of was found two hours later, uninjured, clinging to a hotel-room door.)

Valerie argues that because a baby is completely dependent on his parents for survival, he *has* to be the priority. She says of her son, "Eric's number one in our lives right now because of his needs. And that's hard because we're not number one to each other." She jokingly adds, "Brett can feed himself and change himself. Eric can't." Brett agrees with his wife's assessment of their current priorities. "All my time, when I get home in the evening before he goes to bed, is really devoted to him. So we just don't have the time to fully devote 100% of our attention to each other anymore."

Other parents are not so sure who should come first in the attention pecking order. Loren says, "The love you have for your wife is different from the love you have for your child. And I don't know if one comes ahead of the other. I would like to think that your spouse is always most important." It can be very stressful making sure that everyone gets enough attention. For example, Loren says that when he comes home from work, he notices that he focuses on 17-month-old Lainey first. "As I'm doing that, I'm realizing in my mind the whole time that Stacey is sitting right there, and I don't want her to feel like I'm more interested in Lainey." Stacey is also cognizant of a self-inflicted pressure to give both her spouse and her daughter sufficient attention, especially at the end of Loren's workday. At times she feels as if she is fighting a losing battle. "He comes home from work sometimes, and I'm getting her dinner ready or feeding her. I can't just stop and drop everything ... I just can't help it." It is also hard to ignore a shrieking child. Stacey says, "When Lainey's up and around, and Loren and I are trying to talk, she will want our attention. She'll scream. She doesn't like it when Loren and I try to have an adult conversation."

Closer and closer

The arrival of a first baby often results in a decline in marital satisfaction, particularly for women, but the news is not all grim.[74-76] John Gottman has spent more than a quarter of a century studying marriage, relationships and parenthood, and is one of the most well-regarded researchers in his field. In a 2000 study, he and his colleagues found that couples with a strong marital friendship were less likely to experience a decline in marital satisfaction following the birth of a first child. A woman whose husband expressed fondness and affection for her, and who was aware of what was happening in her life and responded appropriately, was more likely to have a stable or increased level of marital satisfaction. The same was true of a woman who was mindful of what was going on in her husband's life. In contrast, a mother tended to experience a decline in marital satisfaction if her husband criticized her, was disappointed in the marriage, or described their lives as chaotic.[77]

Women experience a greater decline in marital satisfaction following the birth of a first child because they face more physical and emotional demands, assuming more of the housework and childcare responsiblities.[78,79] A father's active participation in caring for the baby can "buffer the decline in marital satisfaction." Not only can it reduce the mother's workload, but it can also reduce her level of stress. And this means she has more time and energy for herself, as well as for her husband. In addition, by becoming more involved in childcare, a father may feel less like an outsider and may gain a better understanding of the challenges that his wife faces in dealing with a newborn.[80]

Many of the men and women interviewed for this book said having a child brought them closer together as a couple by providing them with another point for emotional connection. The birth of their child afforded them an opportunity to forge a new type of partnership as they shared in caring for this tiny person they had just brought into the world. This is consistent with some of Belsky's earlier research, which suggested that as a couple's sense of romance declined after their first child was born, their sense of partnership increased.[81,82]

Jennifer says this is what happened in her marriage: "As far as romance [is concerned], that's definitely suffered." Yet the friendship and partnership Jennifer and Fred have is now stronger. Jennifer describes, "We have something that's intense in common. Like, 'Wow! We did that together.' When [the twins] do something, I can't wait to call him."

For Catherine and Mark, tending to their 1-month-old son, Matthew, has been a true collaborative effort. "I feel there's a real sense of connection now. There's a real sense of teamwork and of a partnership," declares Catherine. She says they have always been homebodies, so having to stay at home with a baby is not a huge change from their pre-baby lifestyle. "We do a lot of projects together around the house, and we work very well like that. However, we don't get to sit and have leisurely conversations like we did before, and sit and watch a television program and then discuss it and have dinner. It's like, 'You eat, and then I'll eat.'"

D.J. says he believes that having a son completed his relationship with Keri. "This will probably sound corny, but I think we're closer now. And yet we were close before. I am extremely fortunate to be married to her," he declares. "I think having Cooper has just made us whole. It's been good. It's been positive. It hasn't been a stressor like I know it is on some families."

Paul makes a similar assessment of his own marriage. "I think we're stronger as a couple. Having Elliot has just added to our family. I mean it certainly hasn't split us in any way. It's made us stronger as a unit. I think there are more stresses in life, generally, finances and constantly worrying that our little boy's OK. ... We still argue. But we used to nit-pick in our younger years when we started going out. We don't do that anymore. You appreciate what you've got more, and those silly little things don't seem as important as they used to. There are more important things to worry about in life."

Paul and Kate have known each other since they were teenagers growing up in Surrey, England. They performed together in school shows. Kate jokes, "I suppose I found him very sexy when we did a show one year and his costume was clingy around his bottom." Of their current relationship, she says, "I think fundamentally we're still the same. Parenthood does get in the way to a certain extent. However, when you share a moment. ... For example, Elliot walked across the room the other day with a Rice Krispies packet on his head, and we both laughed like you wouldn't laugh or feel about anything else. And to share that with someone, both of us would say it's definitely worth it. You do sacrifice a bit, but it's definitely worth it."

Sometimes, when a couple misses what they used to have together, they work that much harder to get it back. After getting caught up in the day-to-day nuances of newborn life, Leslie and Peter made dating a priority again. She says, "We reminded ourselves that this is where it all started. And now we look at William and think, 'Wow! He's a product of that.' You take the relationship back to its roots where you met each other and fell in love with each other. ... You get to do it again. You get to fall in love again because of him, which is really neat." Peter adds, "I think that stems from seeing your partner as much in love with your baby as you are."

Negotiation of time

Because a newborn needs round-the-clock care and attention, it is tough to accomplish in a day what was possible before the baby was born. One pre-baby day is not the equivalent of one postpartum day. And it is not just leisure activities – movies, manicures, golf outings – that get cut from a new parent's schedule. It is even difficult to fit in the basics like eating, sleeping, bathing and going to the bathroom. Time becomes a luxury, a scarce commodity over which couples must constantly haggle. And those negotiations can quickly deteriorate into arguments, given that exhaustion and anxiety have new parents primed for a fight. Consequently, debates over time management become yet another source of tension for new parents.

During the first few months postpartum, Jim and Janine learned the art of negotiation as they each tried to carve out some personal time. Jim describes: "We definitely struggled. She'd say, 'What time is my time?' And once, when it had just been a bad afternoon and I had a hellish day at work – I'm sure every couple struggles with this, you know, you have a bad day at work, and you come home and she dumps the kid off on you – it was like, 'Wait a minute. How is this supposed to work for me? I just spent 12 hours at work with a bunch of crybabies, you might argue, and so did you. But now you're going to get a break, and I have to take over and start this second job?'" Jim and Janine's first few attempts to address this issue were not exactly productive. Jim explains, "We talked through those things, and I would try to get her gift certificates to get a manicure/pedicure or something like that. But as soon as she would go, [the baby] would start screaming, and then whenever she got back, we would both say things that we didn't really mean, and it just separated us even further. I think it made her feel that she couldn't leave him alone with me for fear that he was going to explode, and that I would not know how to handle it. So it was definitely a big, big struggle when he was really a handful for a little while there."

Exacerbating the problem were their unrealistic expectations about just how much time is spent caring for a newborn. Jim admits, "I don't think we realized the time commitment that it was going to take. Just the simple things like going for a run a few days a week for an hour, and some of those little things where you say, 'Oh, I can squeeze an hour here or there,' and, realistically, on some days you just can't." Running is a big deal to Jim and Janine, both marathoners. In fact, at the time of their first interview, they were busy trying to figure out a training/babysitting schedule that would accommodate all their individual practice runs.

Leslie and Peter also make a special effort to accommodate each other. Leslie says, "On the weekends and in the evenings, the moment Peter comes home, he says, 'OK, go exercise, go do something, go finish your emails, go do what you have to do because I know you didn't get to finish those things today.' So he's been very considerate about that kind of thing, and he looks forward to it. He misses William all day long." Peter says, "We were very determined, from the beginning, to make a special effort not to allow children to eliminate what's important to us as individuals, and to continue doing what we need to do. We've made a special effort. Tennis is important to me, and I think I've played more tennis since the baby was born than before. I make a conscious effort to make plans, and I do it in such a way that hopefully it does not interfere with what Leslie needs to do or with the baby."

Loss of couple time

During the postpartum period, many couples actually go through a period of mourning and grieve for the life they used to know. No matter how much a mother and father may love and cherish their new baby, they may sometimes feel as if he is an intruder on their relationship, that he has interrupted the flow and the dynamics of their life together.

After the baby is born, parents have less time and energy to devote to each other. Date nights, leisurely dinners, evenings spent snuggling up in front of the television, even seemingly meaningless small talk, may all seem like distant memories when couples first switch into baby mode. It is a relentless, 24/7 cycle of feeding the baby, changing his diapers, removing the clothes he has just spit up on, putting him to sleep, and soothing him when he cries. There is no downtime to think about what is happening or why it is happening. New parents may feel as if their home has been transformed into a family triage center, where a constant flow of new issues – mainly concerning the baby – must be prioritized and addressed, stat!

Consequently, it is sometimes the most ordinary elements of a couple's life – discussing the day's trivial, mundane events, chatting about a news story, eating dinner together – which are most sorely missed in the first few weeks and months postpartum, for these are the ties that bind. Brett says he and Valerie used to enjoy talking about current events. Now when he sees an interesting story on the news, he must postpone their discussion until "later." "Well, by the time later comes around," says Brett, "I've forgotten about it because I've been focusing my attention on Eric. Normal, small things of the day-to-day relationship go by the wayside. Whereas before, when Eric wasn't around, I had no one else to talk to or pay attention to, so I'd talk to Valerie about her day. I'd ask her how she felt about this and that. I had more time – I know it sounds stupid and small – but I had more time to tell her that I loved her. So I think that the relationship has changed as a result of that."

A couple may find that because they are overwhelmed caring for their new baby and their home, their relationship is depersonalized and becomes almost business-like. Life becomes one big "to-do" list. "It seems so routine," says LeeRan of her life six weeks postpartum. "Tim comes home. We make dinner, get the baby ready for bed, and then it's the end of the night. Tim leaves in the morning and, here I am, by myself again." When asked whether she misses pre-baby life as a couple, LeeRan said, "It gives me this sick feeling. I want our old life back. I just want it to be me and Tim." Alluding to the famous song sung by The Righteous Brothers, and later by Hall and Oates, LeeRan says, "I've been asking Tim, 'Have you lost that loving feeling for me?' He says, 'No, no, no. You're my number one. Not at all.' I feel like he doesn't love me, but I know he does."

In their book *The Seven Principles for Making Marriage Work*,[83] relationship gurus John Gottman and co-author Nan Silver talk about what a couple can do to protect their marriage as they become parents. Gottman and Silver say new parents need to expand their sense of "we-ness" to incorporate their children. They argue that although many "well-meaning experts" suggest that new parents view marriage and family as a balancing act, the two "are not diametrically opposed" but "of one cloth." Occasionally, a couple must have some alone time together. However, new parents should not feel guilty – as many couples do – if they find that they keep coming back to the same topic of conversation: their baby. It is not a sign, as many other marriage experts suggest, that the couple is putting the baby ahead of their relationship, but that together they are adjusting well to parenthood.

Gottman and Silver offer couples a few other tips for staying connected as they "evolve" into parents. They recommend that the mother include the father in caring for the baby, rather than simply telling him what to do or criticizing him when he does not do something *her* way. Because a new mom tends to focus on her baby, she should acknowledge that her partner is still important to her. She needs to let him know that she is still "sensitive" to his needs and that she still has time for the marriage in her busy life. And the father should give the new mother regular breaks away from her newborn so that she can sleep and take care of herself.[83]

Once the baby is born, new parents may find themselves yearning for the spontaneity that used to exist in their relationship. They cannot just decide on a lazy Sunday to head out to the movies and grab a bite to eat. (Speaking of movies, try asking a new parent about any of the Academy Award-nominated movies in theaters the first year after her child's birth. You are not likely to get much of a response!) Everything must be carefully planned and orchestrated, even time for intimacy.

Sex after baby

"It would take Nathan so long to fall asleep, and then we'd both be near tears. ... We definitely weren't in the mood. So I think now that he's getting on to a regular schedule at night, we have more energy at night, and we're both in better moods," says Janine, five months after giving birth to her son. She continues, "We can be a bit more spontaneous than we used to be." In the beginning, Nathan's sleep schedule was too unpredictable for them to take advantage of any free time they might have. They never knew when Nathan might wake up. Jim and Janine's experience is typical. After the baby comes home, the only thing new parents want to do, apart from tending to their child, is sleep. Researchers at the University of Wisconsin, Madison surveyed more than 1,100 men and women found that, on average, parents resumed sexual relations by seven weeks postpartum. By four months postpartum, 90% of parents had engaged in sexual activity.[84]

Numerous factors can contribute to a decrease in sexual activity following the birth of a baby, including fatigue, low energy, fear of another pregnancy and, as Janine mentioned, an unpredictable schedule. A woman may want to avoid sex if she is experiencing pain or tenderness around the site of an episiotomy or cesarean section. Or she may have body image issues, especially if she had unrealistic expectations of walking out of the hospital wearing her pre-pregnancy "skinny" jeans. Consequently, a woman who is upset about her body may lack confidence and feel unattractive. It can take months, even as long as a year, for a woman to lose all of the weight she gained during pregnancy.

Most obstetricians do not even "clear" their patients to have sex until six weeks postpartum. "For some women it's a little earlier, for some women it's a little later, but that's a good ballpark figure," says Dr. Leiter. But the doctor's green light doesn't always mean "go." When Jim did not, as Janine put it, "pounce on her," she questioned whether he was still interested in her sexually. "I was thinking, 'Is it the way I look?' Right away, that's the first thing I thought, 'He's not attracted to me anymore. What's wrong with me?'" Jim says, "In the beginning, maybe the first couple of months, it was a big roadblock in my head. As soon as Nathan was born, I stopped looking at her as my wife and somebody who's very sexual and [instead viewed her as] just Nathan's mom." Jim asserts that he still found Janine physically attractive, but there was "something either emotionally or psychologically that was kind of going on." Janine remarks, "I think that there's something to be said of 'You don't do certain things with moms.'" Not "doing certain things with moms," such as engaging in sexual intercourse, is a belief associated with the Madonna–Whore Complex, which was discussed in Chapter 2.[85] This theory explains how a man may be conflicted about continuing to view his wife, now the mother of his child, as a sexual being.

For Jim and Janine, communicating with each other about what was – or was not – happening in their marriage was a crucial step toward improving their relationship. Janine says, "We knew we weren't right, which was good. And we knew we wanted to be right. That made me feel good." After a two-month-long rough patch, Jim says that whatever issues he had "kind of just faded." Time proved to be a great emotional healer. "I don't know if it was her going back to work and seeing her as not just a mom. All of a sudden, it was like I had my Janine back. She was competitive, she was training [for marathons] again. All of a sudden, it was like, 'Oh, you're not just a mom. You're not just his caregiver. The relationship between you and me is still there.' We just had to adjust it a little bit."

At one year postpartum, Catherine says it is still hard to make the shift from "mommy/caretaker mode to carefree sexual intimacy." "It's a long way to go. You can get there, but it takes time to relax into it, and you never have enough time to do that and spend time together. Quality intimate time just seems to fall off the has-to-get-done list. Everything else is something that gets done as part of getting through the day – meals, changing clothes, bathing, housekeeping, etc. 'Me/Us' becomes optional." Catherine concludes, "Awareness is half the battle. We will find a way to make special time together a priority. It will take effort and commitment, but a healthy and happy marriage is one of the best things you can give your children. So really, taking care of your relationship is just another way of taking care of [your children], too."

The University of Wisconsin study that looked at sexuality during the first year postpartum (as well as during pregnancy) also revealed that at four months postpartum, women who were breastfeeding were significantly less sexually active and experienced less sexual satisfaction than those who were not breastfeeding.[86] A woman who is nursing may believe that because her breasts are now serving a new function – providing nourishment for her baby – they have become desexualized. And she, therefore, views herself as being less sexually attractive.

Some of the women interviewed mentioned that their husbands felt awkward about touching their breasts after seeing them breastfeed. So men, too, begin to see the breasts in something other than a sexual light. Physiological factors also explain why breastfeeding can cause a decrease in sexual activity and/or sexual satisfaction. Breastfeeding can lead to lower estrogen levels, which can cause vaginal dryness, making sex painful for the woman. Valerie says "major dryness" played a role in her diminished sex drive. She also suffered from postpartum depression, which can affect the libido. It has been almost a year since she gave birth, and she and Brett have still not resumed their pre-baby level of physical intimacy. "Oh God, it sucks. I still don't have a sex drive, so it's been really tough for us," acknowledges Valerie, adding, "I was offering 'pity sex,' and after a while my husband said, 'I don't want pity sex.' But I had felt that we needed to be close and that it was important for our marriage." She says they have sex about twice a month, and that she feels "really disconnected" from Brett. Fortunately, they were able to talk about it. "We've had some good conversations. My husband thinks I don't desire him anymore, which doesn't have anything to do with it." But, as Brett sees it, "I would say on my part the desire is certainly there. But I know on her part the desire isn't there."

Men can have a difficult time waiting until their partners are ready to resume sexual relations. After all, Ralph notes that, physically, men are the same as they were before their wives became pregnant. "Nothing's really changed," he says. The Virginia dad took a good-natured approach to being sidelined, commenting, "Nobody warned me about that stuff before I got married. Nobody warned me about it. ... A woman goes through dramatic physical changes during childbirth and pregnancy that can prevent her from having intercourse for a long time. Men don't. Nothing has changed." Like Valerie and Brett, and Jim and Janine, Ralph and Vanessa were able to discuss what had been happening in their relationship. "We joke about it. We talk about it. I don't think it's hard to deal with. I think it's a fact of life. I think as a male you need to be mature, and you need to be ready for that, though," advises Ralph.

Paul says that before he and Kate had Elliot, he worried that the bloody scene in the delivery room would be "horrible and ugly" and that it would "put me off future relations." Paul was happy to report that his fears turned out to be unfounded. When asked if he had conjured up visions of the delivery while having intercourse, Paul answered emphatically, "I can happily say, 'No, no, no.' Thank God!"

Paul admits that it took a while to get back into the swing of things. "I think because it was such a long period of time without anything, it was almost like I had gone back to my virginity. I had to build up the courage again. It was strange. Even though she's my wife and I've been with her for years and years, it was like I had to build up that confidence again, and I almost felt like I had to take her out on dates, and give her a snog and build up to it again. ... I just think it does take a long time to settle back down into a relationship."

Sometimes sex after having a baby is more satisfying and more relaxing. Pre-baby pressure to conceive a child may have detracted from the pleasure of physical intimacy. While they were trying to have a baby, Shannon and Stephen always felt as if they had to schedule sex. They had difficulty conceiving and had five rounds of *in-vitro* fertilization treatments over the course of five years. "Our life together is easier than it was for the five years of infertility," remarks Shannon. "That was constantly looking at the calendar and asking, 'When do we have sex? When do we not have sex? When do I take drugs? When do I not take drugs?' This is actually easier for us. There's not this pressure. ... It's not that we're having sex every night. It's not like we're back to being 20, but it's just easier. When we do it, it's just for fun. It's just to connect with each other. It's not to produce a baby. ... It's just about the two of us again, which is so nice."

For new parents, staying connected is about honoring the marital relationship by creating time and space for their new life as a couple, and as individuals. Couple time can take any number of different forms, including date nights (or lunches), a long walk or jog through the park together, or simply a regularly scheduled time to sit and chat in the comfort of their own home. Ten minutes at the end of the day, after the baby has gone to sleep, to catch up and unwind is like a power nap for relationships. Although not as fulfilling as a full night's sleep, or in this case, a night out on the town, it does have some benefits and is a small but valuable investment in the relationship.

After the birth of a baby, deriving satisfaction from a marriage is about efficiently reorganizing roles and priorities. A successful familial restructuring, in part, hinges on the establishment of an equitable division of household labor and childcare responsibilities. But it is also about tending to the relationship on a regular basis, even when exhaustion renders new parents nearly incapable of expressing a coherent thought.

CHAPTER 8

Perinatal mood disorders and the baby blues

"I was overwhelmed because I didn't know what the hell I was doing. And I was afraid of screwing up my kid. ... Brett would come home and want to know what happened all day. And I'd say, 'Well, I sat on the couch. We nursed. I did this and that.' Days ran together. ... I was just really disconnected from the world ... It was just my son and I going through the motions. ... I was just taking care of his needs but not really doing anything for myself ... I totally forgot about the rest of me. And my role was just that of a mother taking care of her son."

Valerie, a 32-year-old mom from Cleveland, had postpartum depression following the birth of her son, Eric. She says, "I felt guilty that I didn't feel like [his birth] was the best thing that ever happened to me. I mean, yes, I love my son. It's not about that." Before she had Eric, Valerie was a marketing manager in the commercial building products industry. Eventually she returned to the field as a consultant when Eric was one year old. During the first three months postpartum, Valerie was constantly questioning how she could be a successful professional woman responsible for managing others, and, yet, feel incapable of handling one little baby. "I had people reporting to me, who would ask for my advice, who would listen and do the things that I said to do. And now I am faced with this infant who is in total control, and I have no clue what I'm doing. So here's a woman with a master's degree who can't figure out why her kid's crying too much or how to soothe him." She adds, "I went into this thinking, 'I'm educated. I can figure this out.' I remember calling my dad one day and saying, 'I don't know what I'm doing, Dad. That master's degree doesn't mean shit right now.'"

Perinatal mood disorders – those happening around the time of birth – are nothing new. As far back as 400 B.C., Hippocrates was writing about women suffering from mental illness after giving birth. Yet 2,400 years later, we are only just beginning to understand and properly diagnose postpartum depression and the other perinatal mood disorders. In fact, it was not until 1994 that the American Psychiatric Association added depression with a "postpartum onset" – what we more commonly refer to as postpartum depression – to the *Diagnostic and Statistical Manual of Mental Disorders (DSM)*, the bible of psychiatric symptoms and diagnoses.[87] One year after postpartum depression gained "official status" in the United States, more than 22 million television viewers in the U.K. alone watched Princess Diana's famous interview with the

BBC's Martin Bashir, in which she spoke not only of the breakdown of her marriage to Prince Charles, but also about her own struggles with postpartum depression. In that 1995 interview, the princess talked candidly about the onset of her illness after the birth of her son, Prince William in 1982, noting that postpartum depression was a subject that people never discussed. Six years later that would all change.

On June 20, 2001, Houston mother Andrea Yates drowned her five children. Yates had a history of both postpartum depression and postpartum psychosis, a much rarer illness. The media attention garnered by the Houston mother's story helped raise awareness of just how prevalent these illnesses are. However, the media erroneously connected postpartum depression with the killing of children. It is severe cases of postpartum psychosis that have resulted in violent thoughts and, in some instances, infanticide. One to two out of every 1,000 postpartum women experience postpartum psychosis, a break with reality marked by delusional beliefs and hallucinations. A new mother with psychosis may feel as if forces beyond her control are governing her behavior. For example, she may hear voices directing her to harm herself or her infant. Andrea Yates believed that she was a terrible mother and that Satan would torment her children or take them away if she did not kill them. After the Yates tragedy, some women, who otherwise may have sought help for a postpartum mood disorder, instead continued to suffer alone, for fear of being associated with such an unimaginable act. They even worried that their children would be taken from them.

In her first trial, Yates was convicted of first-degree murder, but was ultimately spared the death sentence. Her conviction was later overturned after it was discovered that a prosecution witness gave false testimony. In a dramatic turn of events, a jury found Yates not guilty by reason of insanity when she was retried in June 2006. She has been committed to a state mental hospital.

In addition to the Yates case, the abundance of news stories describing celebrities' battles with postpartum depression has also shed light on this group of mental disorders. Stars such as Brooke Shields, Courtney Cox Arquette and Marie Osmond have all spoken publicly about their personal struggles with postpartum depression – Shields and Osmond both wrote books that became *New York Times* best sellers. Even with all of the information available today, some women who experience symptoms of these illnesses fail to realize that they could be suffering from postpartum depression and are often reluctant to seek help.

The stigma of mental illness continues to exist in our society, despite statistics indicating that more than 18 million adults suffer from some form of depression.[88] There are those who incorrectly maintain that mood disturbances reflect personality defects, and that "strong" people do not get depression. With perinatal mood disorders, there is the additional burden of having a mental illness at a time that is supposed to be filled with joy. A new mother who is not euphoric, who is not experiencing the alleged supreme contentment of womanhood, may feel ashamed. After all, according to the prevailing thinking, how could a "good mother" not be elated by the birth of her child?

Approximately 13% of women who give birth experience postpartum depression.[89] It is crucial for couples to understand the potential risk factors for postpartum depression well in advance of delivery, and to discuss those risks with their obstetrician (or midwife). If the obstetrician is unable to offer this type of assistance, he or she can refer the couple to someone who is trained to deal with perinatal illnesses. Together they can assess the mother-to-be's risks and formulate a plan of action. This plan may include visiting a therapist and/ or talking to a doctor about medication options. It may also involve hiring someone to help with the housework and baby-care responsibilities during the early postpartum period, and finding a support group should the need arise. The group should be specifically geared toward women with postpartum depression, not a garden variety "new moms'" group. For a woman with depression, attending a basic new mothers' group may make her feel uncomfortable or heighten her sense of inadequacy upon seeing other new mothers who seem so elated by their new roles.

Creating a support plan does not guarantee that a woman will be able to avert depression following the birth of her baby. However, it is possible to lessen the severity and duration of symptoms with appropriate interventions during pregnancy or immediately after delivery. The key is early detection, so that a woman can immediately get the help she needs. Once a woman puts these protective measures in place, she will be better equipped to cope with postpartum life. Early detection also enables a woman to get treatment before her depression becomes chronic and resistant to treatment.

Perinatal mood disorders cut across all lines of ethnicity, socio-economic status and even gender. As part of a massive, longitudinal study, a research team led by an Oxford University psychiatrist found that approximately 3.6% of new fathers appeared to be suffering from depression at two months postpartum. These fathers experienced symptoms, including mood swings, and feelings of hopelessness, anxiety and irritability.[90]

A new mother's depression can influence the marital relationship, her developing attachment with her infant, and even her husband's vulnerability to depression.[91,92] One review of studies conducted between 1980 and 2002 identified maternal depression as the strongest predictor of paternal depression in the year following the birth of a child.[93]

The pregnancy blues or postpartum depression?

One major misconception is that the "baby blues" is a mild form of postpartum depression. Although all postpartum mood disorders used to be grouped together under the umbrella of "the blues," postpartum blues is actually considered to be a normal part of postpartum adjustment that as many as 75% of women experience. A variety of factors contribute to the onset of the postpartum blues, including the enormous hormonal shifts that follow birth, the stress of delivery, and the typical new mother anxieties. The blues generally begins within a few days after birth. Symptoms include tearfulness, anxiety, some sadness or irritability, fatigue and difficulty sleeping. The baby blues may last for as little as a few days, and will typically disappear by two to three weeks postpartum, especially if the woman is getting sufficient rest, nourishment and emotional support.

People often confuse the blues with postpartum depression because the two share some of the same symptoms. The difference lies in the severity, duration and timing of the symptoms. Postpartum depression can occur at any time during the first year after the baby's birth, and may last longer than just a few weeks. LeeRan says she cried at least once a day for two to three weeks. When asked six weeks postpartum if she thought she had postpartum depression, she responded, "I don't think so because I don't feel that way anymore. I didn't feel really depressed. I don't know. I think it was more hormonal and being tired and maybe a little depressed. I'm not really sure how to differentiate between the depression and just feeling blue and generally tired." Anyone who believes she (or he), or a partner, may be suffering from postpartum depression should immediately seek advice from a healthcare provider.

The symptoms most commonly experienced by women with postpartum depression are sadness, excessive worry and anxiety, changes in appetite and sleep patterns, overwhelming feelings of hopelessness, guilt and, in some cases, suicidal thoughts. It is not unusual for a woman with postpartum depression to feel emotionally disconnected from her infant. She may also feel frightened about being left alone with her baby, and have serious doubts about her ability to care for him or her. It is normal for a first-time mother to feel apprehensive about her new responsibilities. However, a woman with postpartum depression has an even more pronounced sense of inadequacy. She may feel so incompetent, and so incapable of coping, that she believes that her baby would be better off with another mother. Yet, she may be reluctant to ask for help, fearing others will view this as a sign of weakness and assume that she does not measure up as a parent. Other postpartum illnesses include postpartum obsessive-compulsive disorder, postpartum panic disorder, postpartum stress disorder and postpartum psychosis.

Postpartum thyroiditis is not a mood disorder, but the symptoms – sadness, exhaustion, and difficulty concentrating – mimic those of postpartum depression. Five to ten percent of women who give birth have postpartum thyroiditis, a physiological condition in which the gland that regulates metabolism is either underactive or overactive.[94] A blood test can determine whether a woman has a thyroid problem. Sometimes no treatment is necessary and the condition abates on its own. In other cases, medication or hormone replacement pills are prescribed.

Mood disorders during pregnancy

Because postpartum depression has received so much attention, and because pregnancy is deemed by so many people to be the happiest time in a woman's life, it may come as a surprise to learn that approximately 10% of women are depressed *during* pregnancy.[95] An expectant mother may not suspect that she has antenatal depression (the term "antenatal" means occurring before birth) because some of the symptoms – sleep and appetite disturbances, low sex drive, low energy and fatigue – are similar to the normal physiological effects of pregnancy.

Antenatal anxiety has not been studied nearly as much as antenatal depression, but it is not uncommon.[96] In one study, researchers evaluated approximately 1,700 pregnant women in Northern Sweden and diagnosed almost seven percent with an anxiety disorder.[97] It is crucial to treat any mood disorder during pregnancy, not only for the sake of the mother and her emotional well-being, but also for the sake of her unborn child and his physical health. Antenatal depression, as well as antenatal anxiety, can increase the likelihood that a woman will develop postpartum depression.[98] Furthermore, researchers at the University of California, Irvine found that psychosocial factors (high prenatal stress and low social support) were associated with higher rates of preterm deliveries, and small-for-gestational age and low-birth-weight babies.[99] A premature, low-birth-weight baby is at a greater risk of developing respiratory and heart problems during the newborn period, and will likely need special care in the hospital's neonatal intensive-care unit.

Who is at risk for postpartum mood disorders?

In their book, *Women's Moods: What Every Woman Must Know About Hormones, the Brain, and Emotional Health*,[100] authors Deborah Sichel and Jeanne Watson Driscoll liken a mood disorder to an earthquake. They analogize its onset to a weakened subterranean fault line that "gives way" due to "internal pressures," creating "chaos and destruction above." According to Sichel and Driscoll, a woman has "fault lines" that represent her brain biochemistry, her life events and her hormonal chemistry. When stress and/or changes in hormone levels overwhelm these fault lines, "an emotional earthquake occurs."

There are numerous risk factors for postpartum depression, including a personal or family history of depression (postpartum or otherwise) or anxiety, a history of premenstrual dysphoric disorder (a disturbance in mood associated with the menstrual cycle), and the hormonal changes caused by fertility treatments.[101]

Psychosocial risk factors can also increase a woman's vulnerability to postpartum depression. Sleep deprivation, a complicated pregnancy or delivery, and unexpected health problems with the baby all fall into this psychosocial category. Other risk factors include, a history of physical, mental or sexual abuse and a family or personal history of chemical dependency. In addition, major financial strains and stressful life events – a move, a divorce or a death in the family – can impact a woman's mental health during the postpartum period. Because pregnancy is such a powerful physiological and psychological experience, the long-forgotten pain of other losses, such as a parent's death, can also put a woman at a greater risk of developing depression after childbirth.

Time and again, research confirms that a man's support is crucial to his partner's emotional health during this often stressful period.[102] Shaila Misri, one of the leading reproductive psychiatrists in the field of women's health and perinatal illnesses, has written extensively about mood disorders related to childbirth. In a 2000 study, she and her colleagues found that women with postpartum depression who were supported by their partners exhibited a marked decrease in symptoms.[103] The work of two Australian researchers, Philip Boyce and Anthea Hickey, further emphasized the link between the quality of a couple's relationship and a woman's postpartum psychological state. Their 2005 study showed that a woman has an increased risk of developing postpartum depression if she has a poor relationship with her partner or trouble communicating with him.[104]

Recognizing postpartum depression

Cleveland mother Valerie says she was never officially diagnosed with depression prior to having a baby, but recalls feeling depressed at certain times in her life. She also says that whenever she was menstruating, "I was a crazy woman. Literally, my head would pop off and spin around. I just had these major swings with PMS. And so because I had read somewhere that if you did have significant PMS mood swings you'd be more likely to have postpartum depression, we certainly were watching for it." Valerie was prescribed an antidepressant for her severe mood swings. She stopped taking it once she decided to get pregnant.

Despite watching for signs of postpartum depression, Valerie and Brett were not proactive in taking measures to prevent it. Valerie says, "We were hoping it wasn't going to happen. Isn't that horrible? That was our thought process – 'Maybe it won't happen.'" She continues, "I don't think we noticed it because it creeps up on you. We were looking for one big sign and it wasn't one big thing. I think Zoloft does it the best in the commercial with those stupid little cartoons, the little round ovals. They kind of look gloomy. Everything's just gray. It's not a horrible gray. It's just gray."

Valerie initially thought it was just the normal, post-pregnancy hormonal changes that were making her feel down. She believed she could just ride it out. "You're crying and you're absolutely in love with this creature that you just gave birth to," she says. "You're crying, almost like, 'Oh, this? I can handle this. This makes sense to me. It wasn't the depression. It was just hormone fluctuation.' And I thought, 'Great, we made it through.' And then week three hit, and that's really when it started. ... He hit colic, and that's when I started to feel overwhelmed, I guess. We didn't have family to help us out, so it was just me, my husband and Eric."

Brett says he noticed a change in Valerie after the baby was born. "I observed that she felt melancholy and not really, 'Oh woe is me,' but she just had a careless attitude, and that's not like Valerie," he explains. He says Valerie spoke of feeling like "an island." "She was all alone with Eric, tending to his needs, feeding him and changing him and trying to get him to nap every two to three hours. She just didn't have any time for herself. Simple things that I know she wanted to get done during the day, she just wasn't getting done. ... That also tipped me off."

Two months before Eric was born, Brett's mother died. Three weeks postpartum, Valerie lost her job when her company downsized. "So I was dealing with these changes. My mother-in-law died. We have a son who's colicky and I lose my job, my identity of being this – I don't want to say high-powered exec because I wouldn't call myself that – but this woman in the workforce who is making good money, to now a mom who's clueless."

In addition to feeling disconnected, isolated and overwhelmed, Valerie had what she called "these strange thoughts." She describes them: "This is one thing that I had read about that I did have ... and it's one of the things that made me think I had postpartum depression because I had these bizarre thoughts. I'd be holding my son, and I'd be in the kitchen, and I'd see the knife set that's there in the wood block and think, 'What if I had a knife and I was cutting something, and it slipped and cut my son?' Not that I would pick up a knife and cut my son. It's not that kind of thing going on, just really bizarre thoughts. Or I'd be in the bathroom blow-drying my hair and think, 'What if there was water in the sink, and I dropped the hairdryer in there and I electrocuted myself and I died? Who would take care of Eric? And, meanwhile, he's sleeping in his crib. No one would be home for another six hours.' They were morbid thoughts." Valerie emphasizes that she did not feel any animosity toward her son, nor did she have a desire to harm him. "Most of the thoughts were about situations where I would hurt myself and no one would be there to take care of Eric." Brett eventually convinced Valerie to go to the doctor, a critical step that would put her on the road to recovery.

Treatment

Decisions about treating depression during pregnancy, or in the postpartum period, depend on the symptoms that appear, their severity and their duration. Treatment generally involves the use of antidepressant medications in combination with short-term psychotherapy. Group support can also be effective in alleviating symptoms, by reducing a woman's feelings of isolation, and by helping her to understand that there are other women experiencing the same feelings.

Among the most controversial issues regarding treatment is whether to prescribe medication to a woman who is pregnant or breastfeeding. Doctors need to weigh carefully the risks of leaving a woman's depression untreated against the risks of exposing her baby to potentially harmful drugs. Dr. Shari Lusskin, Director of Reproductive Psychiatry at New York University School of Medicine, says, "We have a lot of data regarding the risks of untreated depression for both the mother and the baby. During pregnancy, [these risks] are low birthweight, premature delivery and obstetrical complications." With severe depression, there is also the risk of suicidal thoughts, or worse.

When a woman discontinues her antidepressants during pregnancy, she runs the risk of having a relapse. "Clearly depression is more common in pregnancy than we had appreciated in the past. Pregnancy itself is not protective [against depression]," says Dr. Catherine Spong, Chief of the Pregnancy and Perinatology Branch at the National Institute of Child Health and Human Development (NICHD). Dr. Spong, who also practices maternal fetal medicine, adds "I do tell patients that it's common to relapse" when they stop taking their antidepressants. A study led by researchers at Massachusetts General Hospital revealed that almost 70% of women who discontinued their antidepressants in early pregnancy, or shortly before conception, had a relapse of depression.[105]*

Elizabeth, a high school teacher living in Kansas, had a history of anxiety and depression. After she became pregnant, her psychiatrist advised her to stop taking one of her antidepressant medications, Trazodone, immediately. She remained on Prozac, but went "cold turkey" with the Trazodone, and her old symptoms returned. "That's when everything went downhill," recalls Elizabeth. Her anxiety returned in full force, and she also experienced symptoms of depression. "For 10 or 11 nights, I went without sleep. My body would not sleep. I was completely overrun with anxiety. ... Day to day, I couldn't function,

---

*Although the researchers who conducted this study are well regarded in the field of perinatal psychiatry, an article published on July 11, 2006 in the *Wall Street Journal* questioned why several authors of the study, including lead author Lee S. Cohen, failed to disclose their financial ties to pharmaceutical companies that manufacture antidepressants. In a response published on July 12, 2006 in the *Journal of the American Medical Association*, Dr. Cohen and colleagues said that they did not view their associations as relevant to the study because it was "a federally funded prospective observational study in which patients independently decided" whether to stay on medication. All the participants received the same educational information describing the potential risks of prenatal exposure to antidepressants and of untreated depression in pregnancy. Furthermore, the response states that the study did not look specifically at any one drug. Dr. Cohen and his colleagues concluded that they regretted not disclosing the financial ties of all the authors, and acknowledged, "Such disclosures would have provided utmost transparency with respect to potential conflict of interest." The *Journal of the American Medical Association* responded by tightening its conflict-of-interest policy.

and I was just completely overwhelmed. And I kept thinking, "If I can't take care of myself now, how am I ever going to take care of my baby when my baby comes?" During the time she was not taking Trazodone, Elizabeth's symptoms became so severe that she considered terminating the pregnancy, but instead she decided to take control of her illness. Elizabeth flew halfway across the country to the Women's Mental Health Program at Emory University, where some of the country's leading researchers are studying treatments for perinatal mood disorders. She was diagnosed with generalized anxiety disorder. The doctors at Emory put her on a low dose of Trazodone and kept her on the Prozac. Her mood stabilized, and she began to feel a connection with her baby by the beginning of the second trimester. Elizabeth says the doctors at Emory convinced her that it was safe to take medicine while she was pregnant and adds, "They instilled in my mind that healthy women have healthy babies." Eventually, Elizabeth gave birth to a healthy little girl named Liza.

Postpartum depression can affect the quality of a mother's developing relationship with her baby. A new mother with depression may feel withdrawn or emotionally detached from her infant. Postpartum depression can affect her capacity to respond in a consistent manner when her baby needs her. In contrast, a mother who is attuned to her baby's needs, and addresses them, teaches her infant that people will respond when he requires their attention. She also shows him that he is worthy of that attention. In essence, she teaches him about trust. When a mother's depression interferes with her ability to connect with her infant, that can detrimentally affect her child down the road. Research has shown that children of mothers who are postnatally depressed are at greater risk for cognitive, behavioral and emotional developmental problems.[106,107]

The need for continued treatment of depression during pregnancy and in the postpartum period is beyond dispute. One of the most effective means of treating depression is with medication, notably the class of antidepressants known as selective serotonin reuptake inhibitors (SSRIs), which include the drugs Prozac, Paxil and Zoloft. But a woman who is pregnant or breastfeeding exposes her baby to any medication she takes. Therefore, the obvious question becomes: Is the medication dangerous for the baby?

Dr. Gideon Koren is the founder and director of The Motherisk Program at The Hospital for Sick Children in Toronto. For more than 20 years, the Motherisk team has been focusing on maternal-fetal toxicology, and counseling women on and researching the risks of various medicines. Dr. Koren says that over the past 15 years, we have accumulated a large number of studies on the effects of a baby being exposed in utero to SSRIs. "In general, it does not appear that they increase, in any clinically significant way, the risk for birth defects," he notes, continuing, "A smaller number of studies continued to follow these kids up for neuropsychological development. And, again, they did not show (an increase in adverse) effects compared with control groups."

However, results released from three recent studies indicate an increased risk of a few serious defects. Further research is needed to confirm the results and to better prove causation – that the defects were, indeed, caused by the medicines and not by other independent factors. Preliminary results from two studies suggest a higher incidence of heart defects in babies who were exposed to Paxil *in utero* early in pregnancy.[108–110]* In these studies, researchers relied on information that was self-reported to a national birth registry and to an insurance claims database. The criticism of this data-gathering method is that it is dependent on what people choose to report.

"You don't always get a very representative sample of the population," says the NICHD'S Dr. Spong. She adds, "A lot of times people will be exposed to medications in pregnancy, and they won't have one of these complications. And so then it's never reported in any of these registries or in any of the studies. That's the inherent difficulty in all of this – that when nothing happens, nothing goes wrong, that's rarely reported." But Dr. Spong says that despite the drawbacks of this data-collecting method, one should not discount the results of the two Paxil studies. "It's still information, and I think all information is good and is important for someone to consider."

Dr. Christina Chambers, a researcher from the University of California, San Diego, published a study in 2006 showing that the incidence of a potentially fatal breathing problem called persistent pulmonary hypertension of the newborn (PPHN) was six times higher in babies who had been exposed to SSRIs *in utero* in late pregnancy. To put these figures in perspective, PPHN usually occurs in about 1 or 2 in 1,000 babies. In the Chambers study, the rate was 6 to 12 in 1,000 infants. In addition, Dr. Chambers, like the Paxil researchers, did not use a random sample. She identified 377 women who had babies with PPHN and compared them with a group of women who had normal, healthy babies.[111]

Dr. Koren says, "The only thing we know for sure that the SSRIs do after birth is the withdrawal syndrome, and that's not surprising." He says that just like adults who stop taking SSRIs "cold turkey," babies may also exhibit signs of withdrawal (after they are born). One Israeli study published in 2006 found that a third of babies exposed to their mothers' SSRIs *in utero* exhibited withdrawal symptoms, including high-pitched crying, tremors, gastrointestinal problems and disturbed sleep.[112]

Regarding infant exposure to antidepressants through breastfeeding, "all SSRIs are secreted into breast milk."[113] Research on some of the most popular SSRIs, including Zoloft, shows that only very low levels of these drugs have been found in the bloodstreams of breastfed babies.[114] Because the research

---

*One study which looked at Swedish national registry data cited a twofold increase in cardiac defects. The rate was 2% among those infants who were exposed to Paxil in early pregnancy, compared with 1% among all registry infants. The second study, sponsored by Glaxo-SmithKline, the manufacturer of Paxil, found that the rate of cardiac malformations was 1.5% for infants exposed in the first trimester, compared with 1% for infants exposed to other antidepressants.

on infants' exposure to antidepressants through breastfeeding is limited to case reports and small studies, further study is needed.[115] There have been a few case reports of seizures and colic in infants whose mothers took SSRIs while breastfeeding, but a case report is an individual incident.[116] "That's not proof of increased risk," says Dr. Koren, adding, "No study yet has shown adverse effects" due to a mother exposing her baby to these medicines via breast milk.

The U.S. Food and Drug Administration (FDA) categorizes these drugs for use during pregnancy. However, reference manuals such as Thomas Hale's *Medications and Mothers' Milk*[117] and Gerald Briggs' *Drugs in Pregnancy and Lactation*[118] (co-authored with Roger Freeman and Sumner Yaffe), offer far more detailed information on what the latest studies indicate regarding the risks (to an infant) associated with a mother's use of antidepressants during pregnancy and/or breastfeeding. References such as these have become invaluable resources for physicians.

When Valerie finally decided to visit her physician, she was given a series of blood tests to rule out any physical condition that might be responsible for her symptoms. Valerie says that afterwards, "I brought up the postpartum depression and just burst into tears. And that's the first time I cried about it." The doctor proposed prescribing antidepressants. Valerie was concerned about taking medicine while she was breastfeeding, so Brett joined her at the doctor's office, along with Eric's pediatrician, to discuss the issue. Together, they decided that Valerie would take Lexapro, a drug commonly prescribed for depression and anxiety. Valerie's doctor told them that it was generally considered safe to use while breastfeeding. Valerie says one of the reasons she chose to take medicine was because "If you feel better, then your child will feel better, too."

Of her initial reluctance to seek medical attention, Valerie explains: "Depression is a funny thing. One day you're like, 'Oh man, I'm calling the doctor tomorrow. It was a long day and I just feel like a big blob.' And then the next day you have a little energy, and you do some more things and you think, 'Oh, I feel fine.' And then the next day you're a big blob again. And that's what really screws with you because sometimes you feel like you have control of it and then you don't."

Valerie says that once the medicine kicked in, "It was like two new people. Eric [coincidentally] wasn't as colicky, and I was more engaged. I had energy. I could do 12 things a day like I used to." And she was finally able to take care of herself. Valerie joined a lactation group at her local hospital to meet and talk with other moms because she had found motherhood isolating. "I reached out because I did feel like an island," notes Valerie. "I think part of it was that the postpartum depression was keeping me from reaching out earlier." The mothers' group "made her sane," especially listening to other mothers' war stories. "It was just nice to get advice from other moms, or just to say, 'Oh yeah, I've been there.' ... Sometimes you'd hear a worse story than yours, like, 'Oh, your child got up nine times last night! Mine got up only three times. That makes me feel better!' "

Shannon was diagnosed with postpartum depression about three weeks after giving birth to twins, and was prescribed the antidepressant Zoloft. Like Valerie, she debated whether to take medication while breastfeeding and eventually decided that it would be the right course of action for her. "I was just so depressed that I kept thinking, 'It's better for my boys for me not to be depressed than it is for me not to take this medicine.' ... Being a proactive person, I don't like to feel bad. And I didn't want the boys to see me feeling bad, even though they were so young." She continues, "I wanted to be happy about them, and I wanted to be happy about the whole situation. So whatever I could do proactively to make us all happy, then I was OK with that."

Shannon says that, prior to starting the medication, "I never felt like hurting the babies, which I am really grateful about. I just felt overwhelmed, and I just wanted someone else to come in and take care of us. I just wanted someone to let me sleep for a few hours, that kind of thing. If Stephen could have quit his job and been home with me every day of the week, I think my postpartum depression would've been fine." She found herself frequently crying uncontrollably. "I remember my mother-in-law wanted to visit, and she wanted to come in the late afternoon. And I actually thought to myself, 'Oh my gosh! I cry at five o'clock every day. I can't have her come then.'"

Coping

Shannon and Stephen recruited friends, family members and professionals to help them manage the enormous workload of caring for twins. For a week, Shannon's father made the one-hour commute to her house to lend a hand. "He stayed all day long, and he did our laundry. I was in the full swing of postpartum depression. I was crying all day long, and he would just take care of the boys for me, let me go take a nap. ... He was great. He did everything. He would take care of both boys, change their diapers, feed the two of them. I never would have thought that my dad could do that." Stephen notes that employing a night-nanny service one night a week was also a blessing.

Shannon says the instructor who taught her birthing class urged people not to be shy about asking for help. The teacher, herself a mother of twins, even recommended that couples put up a white erase-board on the refrigerator to list everything they need, so that family and friends could handle the new parents' requests for help. "Everybody just automatically assumes they should say, 'Oh, I'm fine. I don't need anything.' But she said tell them what you need. If you need a spaghetti dinner, you need that. If you need four loads of laundry done, that's what it is. So I tried to be cognizant of that," notes Shannon. Although she never ended up purchasing an erase-board, she did rely on others for help. Members from her church kept Shannon's kitchen pantry well stocked. People brought Shannon and Stephen enough food to last almost five weeks. "We literally didn't cook. At some point it just felt like we had too much food, so people would say, 'I really want to bring something. What can I bring?' And so I would say, 'Well, bring a case of bottled water.' It was so amazing."

Elizabeth, who suffered from anxiety while pregnant, went to great lengths to ease the stress and chaos of the postpartum period. During her pregnancy, she joined a support group for mothers with postpartum depression because she was unable to find a group for women with antenatal depression/anxiety. Her group talked about managing time efficiently during the postpartum period and introduced her to the concept of a doula. "I had a doula come in three days a week, which was so helpful. She would just come in and keep Liza company, and I would go upstairs and sleep some days. Other days, she'd go to the grocery store or do whatever else I needed her to do." Elizabeth and her husband, Brian, also staggered their visitors for the first six weeks so that there was always someone around to help. Her planning paid off. Although she experienced some anxiety after Liza was born, Elizabeth believes that she would have been a lot worse had she not been taking antidepressants and had she not put a support network in place. Most importantly, she was able to enjoy her new baby daughter.

The father's role

Valerie gives Brett all of the credit for convincing her to seek help for her postpartum depression. Everyday he would come home from work and ask how she was feeling. "He was watching for [postpartum depression], but didn't really know what to look for. It just creeps up on you," explains Valerie. Men are frequently the first line of defense for women facing postpartum depression. Often, a man knows his wife or partner better than anyone else, and is in the best position to observe any shifts in mood or behavior.

Expectant and new fathers should become familiar with the primary symptoms of postpartum depression, either by speaking with a healthcare provider or by reading up on the subject so that they know what to look for. When Stephen spoke to the nurses at the hospital, they suggested that he observe his wife to see whether she was crying a lot, did not feel like getting out of bed, or had a desire to hurt her boys. He explains, "As a guy, I wanted to fix things. But there's nothing I could have said that would have fixed [her postpartum depression]." When asked what advice he had for other men whose partners might have postpartum depression, he said, "Just try to encourage her to talk to someone, such as a doctor. Definitely be there to listen to her."

Sometimes, in an effort to be positive and helpful, men will offer well-intentioned words of wisdom that, for some women, end up sounding insulting or condescending. Examples include: "Focus on the things you have to feel happy about," "Think positive," "What have you got to be depressed about? You just had a new baby," or a particular favorite – "You can snap out of this." Well, if she could merely "snap out of it," wouldn't she have done so already? After all, no one enjoys feeling depressed.

Most women realize that their husbands cannot "fix" their postpartum depression. Usually, a woman just wants someone to talk to so that she does not feel so frightened or alone with her illness. A mother experiencing a postpartum mood disorder may be irritable and particularly sensitive, and so she may lash out at those around her. As in the labor and delivery room, women tend to yell at the people with whom they feel safest, typically their significant others. Men should try not to take this personally, but it is acceptable to set limits. Men do not have to be emotional punching bags.

So what *should* a man say when the woman he loves is suffering from postpartum depression? Simple words of support and encouragement tend to have the most meaningful impact: "We will get through this," "I am not going to let you go through this alone," "This is temporary. I know you will get better," "This is not your fault. You have not done anything wrong," and "You are a great mom. I love you."

A new dad can help his partner in a number of other ways as well. He can arrange for her to have a solid block of time to sleep, by providing time for naps or by handling the night feedings. Or he can get a baby nurse, doula, friend or relative to handle these tasks. He can also persuade her to lower her expectations regarding the upkeep of the house, as well as other responsibilities not directly related to caring for herself and the baby. If either of them is bothered by the idea of a messy house, the father can hire help or enlist a willing relative or friend to pick up the slack.

Finally, men need to take care of themselves so that they are better able to support their wives both physically and emotionally. That self-care means getting adequate rest and reserving even just a couple of hours a week to continue an activity they enjoy, be it playing poker with the guys, watching a game on television or playing golf. Postpartum mood disorders can affect the whole family. So on some level, each member of the family must be cared for and supported.

CHAPTER 9

The many paths to parenthood

Today there are more ways than ever to put together a family. We have variations aplenty of the traditional male–female, love-marriage-then-the-baby-carriage scenario: same-sex parents, heterosexual unmarried parents, and stay-at-home dads. In addition, a fair number of single, educated women in their late thirties and early forties are choosing to have children to add to their already rich, but partnerless lives. This chapter takes a look at the different ways families come to be, and the unique stresses and issues associated with each path to parenthood.

Adoption

"The way I want to explain it to him one day is that God meant for him to be with us all along, and that this was just the path we had to take in order to get him," says Pam, a mother from Atlanta. She and her husband adopted their son, Jeoffrey, when he was 4 weeks old. Pam and her husband (also named Jeoffrey) had been trying to have a baby for five years before they opted for adoption. They were going to try *in-vitro* fertilization, but Pam found that complications from fibroid tumors, as well as her chaotic schedule as a flight attendant, made arranging the necessary procedures quite difficult. Yet, she was determined to become a mother. She explains, "I knew that I was going to be a mother, somehow. I'm one of those people who, if I put my mind to something, it's going to happen."

Between 118,000 and 127,000 children are adopted each year in the United States.[119] Although some people on the parenting track view adoption as the choice of last resort, their attitudes often change once a little baby is placed in their arms, officially making them parents. Dina Rosenfeld, Director of New York University's Undergraduate Social Work Program, has spent the past two decades studying and consulting on adoptions. She has met with approximately 10,000 families. "I have to tell you that the single most moving thing for me, that I keep hearing over and over again, is that there are no questions in these people's [the adoptive parents'] minds that these were the right children for them, that it was meant to be," says Rosenfeld. This was certainly the case with Pam's adoption. Pam says, "I couldn't have asked for anything more from a birth child than what I received from him."

Pam counts herself lucky. The whole adoption process happened fairly quickly, she believes, because they are an African-American couple who wanted an African-American baby. She had to wait only two months before adopting little Jeoffrey. In contrast, it can sometimes take years to adopt a healthy, white baby. Furthermore, adoptive parents-to-be often must wade through a bureaucratic quagmire, filling out reams of paperwork and dealing with dozens of state and agency officials, and in the case of international adoptions, immigration authorities as well. These future mothers and fathers may also experience heartache on the road to parenthood if their arrangements fall through.

For a pregnant couple, the nine months of physical gestation are also a time of psychological gestation during which feelings about impending parenthood start to surface. Adoptive parents have their own parallel psychological transition period. "I think in some ways the gestational period is paperwork. It's getting all of the different bodies involved to approve you," notes Rosenfeld. One adoptive mom said that after she received a picture of the little baby she was about to adopt from Colombia, she brought the photo to her parents' 50th wedding anniversary party and held it up so that he could be included in the family photo. To her, he was already a part of the family. She had proof that she was about to become a mother, and she had already begun to see herself in that role.

Certain issues can arise when a couple decides to build a family with a son or daughter who is not their biological child. They may grieve over the birth child they were unable to have. They may also feel as if their bodies have failed them, by denying them the chance to accomplish what may seem so natural and automatic for most other people: the creation of a child who is their own flesh and blood. Rosenfeld notes, "I think for some people, they have never gotten over the fact that they have not gotten pregnant and have not had a birth child, even though they are obviously parents. For other people, the fact that they have become parents [means that] the whole sort of nightmare of fertility treatments has really been put behind them, and it's relieving. So often, once people become parents and have loved parenting, the only part they can't understand is why they stayed so long in that infertility world."

Sometimes adoptive parents have trouble accepting that their adopted child "belongs" with them, that they are his real parents. They may also worry about bonding with their child. But the bonding process is the same for all parents of newborns, at least in the sense that it is about parents getting to know their baby, and the baby getting to know them.

Those who adopt should be prepared to deal with some inappropriate comments and questions. Some adoptive parents are asked about the cost of the adoption, as if they had just bought a sofa. Adoptive parents may also find themselves fielding questions about the birth mother's circumstances. "It's amazing the insensitive questions that people can ask, such as, 'Oh, was the mother on drugs?'" remarks Pam. Rosenfeld advises adoptive parents to view these comments and questions as educational opportunities: "These people are saying these things to you, not because they want to hurt you or because they're mean, but just because they don't know."

Over the past decade, we have seen a trend toward open adoption. Open adoption allows for some form of contact between the biological mother and the adoptive family, both during the pregnancy and after the birth. The degree of "openness" varies widely. Some families simply exchange pictures and letters but never actually meet in person. Others get together regularly. Certain emotions can arise when an adoptive parent and a birth parent are allowed into each other's lives. Adoptive parents may feel guilty about causing the biological mother great pain and grief after adopting her child, or they may come to resent the presence of the birth mother in their lives.

Many adoptive parents struggle with the question of when and how to tell their children that they are adopted, or even whether to tell them at all. Rosenfeld says it is appropriate to disclose this fact "from the very beginning." She adds, "The reason that you do it as early as possible is because you don't want to get into a situation where you have to sit down with your child and say, 'I have something to tell you.' That's not where you want to be. You want to be where it's just a natural part of a child's life. So, for example, they would be able to say, 'I'm from New York, I'm Catholic, I'm adopted, I have two sisters.'" Rosenfeld continues, "It's not a conversation stopper, it's not something to be embarrassed about, and it's also not something to go around telling everyone. It just is. And the reason why I push for talking about it very early is because although the children have no idea what you're talking about for a long time, it helps parents become comfortable with the topic. Also, the parents don't sit around and worry about how they are going to bring it up, and when and who's going to bring it up."

Fertility treatments

In vitro is Latin for "in glass." Taken literally, *in-vitro* fertilization (IVF) implies fertilization in a glass test tube, although these days the process takes place in a petri dish. Dr. Patrick Steptoe and Dr. Robert Edwards created the first "test-tube baby," Louise Brown, in England in 1978. Three years later, the first successful IVF procedure was performed in the United States. Since 1978, more than three million babies have been born worldwide via IVF and other assisted reproductive technologies.[120] This total does not include babies born to mothers who underwent simpler fertility procedures, such as intrauterine insemination (IUI), or who took fertility medications or hormones.

The IVF process begins with the woman taking fertility drugs to stimulate egg production. Doctors then extract the eggs and fertilize them with the man's sperm in a petri dish. Three to five days later, embryos are transferred to the uterus. About two weeks after that, the woman takes a pregnancy test. The likelihood of multiple births is high, given that more than one embryo is typically inserted.

Nearly one in six couples is infertile.[121] A couple is deemed infertile if they have been unable to conceive after having unprotected sex regularly for a year. In five years, Shannon and Stephen went through three IUI treatments, five IVF treatments and one miscarriage before Shannon became pregnant with the twins, who would eventually be known as Nate and Owen. "It was really rough," remarks Stephen. It was especially difficult for Shannon and Stephen to watch their siblings and friends with their own children. Shannon and Stephen were married for five years before they started trying to have a child. "The first five we weren't trying, and everybody's looking at us like, 'Why don't you have kids?' And then while we were trying, it made it even more difficult because people would say, 'Why did you wait? You should've had them when you were younger,'" says Stephen.

Shannon describes what those five years of hopes and disappointments were like:

> "It was harder for me in the first part of the five years than it was toward the end, which sounds funny. You'd think it would build up to a crescendo. But in the beginning, I was just distraught over not being able to achieve something I thought I should be able to achieve. You think, 'OK, if I work really hard, I can go to college. If I work really hard, I can go to grad school. I can take out loans. I can pay them off. I can be diligent.' You sort of make your future. And this was sort of the first thing that I couldn't make happen, no matter how hard I tried."

Shannon notes that, later, she went through a "whole religious thing." "I felt like, 'How can God let people who do crack have babies, and he won't let me have a baby?' I was just feeling angry at all that and angry at the world and angry at everyone who could have a child. And that would kind of ebb and flow over the course of time," she remembers. "By the time we were doing our last IVF, I was kind of OK with it. I was feeling really good about adoption. I was feeling like maybe that's what we were meant to do and that life was pretty great. Even though I couldn't get pregnant, I could still be an OK person, that it didn't have to do with my self-worth. It took me a long time to get there."

As Shannon and Stephen began to explore adoption, their twins were conceived. They received the good news while shopping for reindeer plates in *Pottery Barn*. "From there, I called my mother and Stephen's mother. We called just about everybody who knew that we had been going through the IVF. We were just so happy. And I just knew that this one was a keeper." Compared with the previous five years of fertility treatments, the pregnancy was a breeze, especially after the first trimester of morning sickness. "From then on, it was great – the whole thing – happy, healthy," exclaims Shannon. At 37 weeks, twins Nathan and Owen were born.

The process of trying to get pregnant can be stressful for any couple, let alone one with fertility issues. Scheduling sex can be a chore. Then there is the cost of fertility treatments, which can be quite a financial strain if they are not covered by insurance. Fortunately, Shannon and Stephen live in Massachusetts, a state that requires insurance companies to cover the costs of fertility treatments regarded as "medically necessary." Their insurance company covered all five IVF treatments, which cost $10,000 per cycle.

Single moms

Single mother Renee remembers attending a class for expectant parents and being surrounded by couples. "It was so awkward," she explains. "I was listening to all their fears. Mine were so different compared with theirs. Mine were basically, 'Can I do this on my own? What happens if he gets sick, and I have to go to work? Will I lose my job because I'm on my own?' ... Watching them, in a lot of ways, I was kind of jealous because they have each other, and I didn't have that." Renee also worried about how she would manage on a daily basis, how she would take a shower or vacuum the house when there was no one else to watch her son. She found herself gravitating toward single mothers "because they could relate to what my fears were because they were already going through it."

In 2003, the number of unmarried women having babies rose to the highest level recorded in more than six decades. At the same time, the number of unmarried teenagers having children fell for the 12th straight year "to another historic low."[122] More and more single women, especially those who have already established their careers, are *choosing* to start families on their own. The general birth rates for women aged 30 to 44 increased to levels not seen since the 1960s.[123]

Single need not mean alone. The key to having a baby solo, whether by choice or not, is to develop a solid social network. To borrow from the old African proverb popularized by Hillary Clinton, "It takes a village to raise a child." Renee's support network consisted of other single mothers, her friends and her mother – who was also a single mom. Renee says, "I have one girlfriend who is a single mother herself – six kids and four grandbabies. She's been my greatest support. The women I have in my life are very strong. That makes me feel like I can do it. They're not dependent." Support groups for single mothers can show women how to navigate the specific stresses that come with having a baby and raising a child without a partner, such as managing the financial burden and finding back-up childcare.

Twenty-five years ago, psychotherapist Jane Mattes founded the organization Single Mothers By Choice, after she accidentally became pregnant and decided she wanted to be a single mom. She says a single mother needs to mourn the life she expected to have and did not – the life with the big fancy wedding, the house with the white picket fence, and then children. "In order to move on to another plan, it's really a good idea to grieve that dream ... to really acknowledge that there is a loss" and to acknowledge that the events of her life will not occur in the order she had expected, advises Mattes. She continues, "They can still have a husband in their plans, but not in 'the natural order of things.'" Mattes says much of this grieving usually takes place before a single woman determines that she actually wants to move forward with her plans to become a mother.

Renee is a single parent by choice. At the age of 42, she had been dating a man for five years when she decided that she wanted a child. She told him that she wanted to stop her birth control pill so she could get pregnant. Renee says he was not interested in being a parent to her child. So she chose to go it alone. "I made a choice, a conscious decision that that was what I was going to do. I had a house, a job. I worked in a doctor's office as a medical assistant. I was secure. I wanted a family. Finding a mate in my situation was really difficult. As you get older, it's hard to find a mate who doesn't already have children, or have a lot of issues in his life. So this was my choice. I knew this was going to be mine, my baby. I wouldn't have to deal with the father."

One of the advantages of parenting solo – assuming that the father does not want to be involved in the child's life – is that a woman does not have to negotiate with anyone else about how to raise her child. Mattes says, "The good part is that you don't have to worry about compromising more than you might feel comfortable comprising. In fact, you don't have to compromise at all." She says the downside of being a single mom is not having the input of another person, not having a sounding board. This is why it is so important to have a solid support network.

For single women like Renee, parenting is not about having a partner but about providing children with the intangible things that help them to thrive. "It's really about giving them love and trying to do the best that you can to support and guide them. That to me is motherhood."

Stay-at-home dads

"It's a lot less stress than my job before, that's for sure. I'd say the hours are longer. I don't get that much sleep because I'm getting up at night to do one of the feedings. ... At first it was all new and exciting, but I guess some of the luster has worn off. But it's still a lot of fun to spend time with [my son]," says 41-year-old Duke, a stay-at-home dad living in Boulder, Colorado. Before Duke's wife, Dana, got pregnant, the couple decided that Duke would be the primary caregiver. As a facilities planner for the Colorado National Guard, Duke says he was making "a lot less money" than Dana, an attorney, and had a long commute to work.

Dana explains, "We both had agreed that we didn't want to have a child in day care, but I still wanted to have my career, and Duke was excited about staying home." Duke says that even though he is not getting paid to care for Dasam, "To me this is a job ... so I don't see it as being that much of a transition from the outside work world." The only thing he really misses about his old job is the intellectual stimulation. But Duke says he is able to get some of that stimulation from a part-time job with the National Guard. He works one weekend a month, plus a few other times during the year. Of his decision, Duke says, "I'm pretty comfortable staying at home, doing housework, all that kind of stuff."

Duke attends a new *moms'* group with his son, Dasam. "It's a little bit strange. At first I felt a little bit awkward." Duke says that judging by their body language, the women in the group were not too sure what to make of him. "I don't think that I have quite the same connection with them. It seems like the folks in there get along with one another probably a little bit better than I do."

Duke says his friends and family members have been positive about his decision to stay at home with Dasam. Yet, like the women in his new moms' group, they have sometimes conveyed more information with their body language. "When I first tell people, it's obvious that it's not the answer they were expecting to hear."

Hogan Hilling, author of *The Man Who Would Be Dad*,[124] and father of three, is a stay-at-home dad. He says people today are generally more accepting of stay-at-home dads than they were 15 years ago, when he first became his children's primary caregiver. Nevertheless, he urges dads to take the initiative if they hope to be welcomed into the new mother circuit that operates at the playground, playdates and parenting groups. "I've talked to stay-at-home dads and I've said, 'Look, you have to remember that these moms have never had a guy show up before. It's your responsibility as a stay-at-home dad to show these moms that you can be trusted," advises Hilling. "I remember the first time I went to the playground. With all the comments I had heard about women wanting to see dads get more involved, I showed up at the playground thinking they would embrace me." Suffice it to say, no one went out of her way to save him an empty swing. "I couldn't figure it out. I felt really alienated, and wondered, 'What's going on here?' And then I realized that a lot of it had to do with how I presented myself." Hilling says the mothers sensed that he felt uncomfortable stepping into this mom-dominated arena. So he had to make the first move. Hilling explains: "I had to work harder to smile and to be energetic. And then I would have to make comments that normally men don't make, such as, 'Oh, is that your daughter over there? I really like her dress.' ... I had to develop a new comfort mode that would help the moms realize that I really wanted to be there. And once I started doing that, the moms were much more receptive."

There is no accurate statistic indicating just how many fathers are staying at home with their children. Although the latest U.S. Census Data puts the figure at 143,000, the number of stay-at-home dads is probably under-reported.[125]

First, there is confusion about who qualifies as a stay-at-home dad. How many hours per week does a father need to spend with his children in order to call himself a stay-at-home dad? Hilling says a second reason the number from the U.S. Census Bureau may be inaccurate is that many of these dads are still sensitive about their status and, therefore, may be reluctant to report it: "There's a running joke that a lot of stay-at-home dads are afraid to come out of the pantry." Hilling adds, "There's a self-esteem issue because you have to feel pretty darn good about yourself to make this decision and then, not only to make it, but to stick with it."

Developing a healthy acceptance of the stay-at-home dad role may entail learning how to respond effectively to the inevitable barbs about being *Mr. Mom* (a reference to the 23-year-old Michael Keaton movie). Many stay-at-home dads loathe the comparison. After all, the whole comedic premise of the movie was based on the incompetence of Keaton's character. Today's stay-at-home dads are a far cry from Keaton's domestically-challenged Jack Butler. Today's stay-at-home dads are becoming masters of their own domains.

So far, for Duke and Dana, the arrangement is working well. Dana remarks, "There are many days that I wish I was staying home, but there are also a lot of days that I'm thinking, 'Whew, I'm glad that I'm out and about'. I don't feel tethered to home and it feels like a really good balance." And Duke concludes, "I think it's just as important as what I was doing before."

Same-sex parenting

"I think the advantage that homosexual couples have over heterosexual couples is that they did have to put a lot of thought into acquiring a child. There are no accidents in this community. The lesbian mother doesn't come home and say, 'Oh my God, I missed my period,'" remarks Jane Drucker, a marriage, family and child counselor and the author of *Lesbian and Gay Families Speak Out: Understanding the Joys and Challenges of Diverse Family Life*.[126]

In the United States, a third of lesbian couples and a fifth of gay couples have children.[127] During the journey to parenthood, these couples face many of the same issues as their heterosexual counterparts, including shifts in family dynamics, struggles to balance competing roles, loss of couple time, added financial pressures, and complications arising from the new baby division of labor. But, gay and lesbian couples must also contend with a unique set of cultural and legal issues. Front and center has been the debate over same-sex marriages. "One of the reasons why the gay and lesbian community is fighting so hard for marriage is because one of the functions of marriage is that both married partners can be the legal parents of any children of the family," notes Drucker. Absent the recognition of gay marriage (with the exception in the United States of the state of Massachusetts which does allow same-sex marriages) it is difficult to ensure that both parents will have legal guardianship rights should they decide to break up down the road. Adoption laws for same-sex couples vary from state to state and from country to country. Some ban gay and lesbian adoptions altogether, some permit one individual to adopt, while others let both partners adopt.

Drucker advises same-sex couples who are considering parenthood to talk to a family lawyer. An attorney can help them hammer out custody and support issues should the partners decide to separate. Having such an arrangement in place can be especially important if only one parent has legal parental rights. Angela and Jackie live in Coral Springs, Florida. Under Florida law, only Jackie, the biological mother, would be entitled to legal custody of their son, Adam, if the two women decided to end their relationship. But when Jackie was pregnant, she and Angela worked with an attorney and determined that if they decided to end their relationship, Angela would share custody with Jackie, and she (Angela) would be financially responsible for Adam until he reached the age of 18.

Gay couples commonly become parents via surrogacy or adoption. Lesbian couples can also go the adoption route. If a lesbian couple wants a biological child, they will typically use a sperm donor, either getting someone they know to donate the sperm or going through a sperm bank. Jackie had intrauterine insemination (IUI) with sperm from a sperm bank. It was important to her and Angela that they have as much medical background information on the donor as possible. Angela says they did a lot of preliminary research online to find out how the various sperm banks operate and screen candidates. They narrowed it down to one company which, according to Angela, "had a very good background database on the donor, his parents, grandparents, siblings and aunts and uncles, as far back as they could go."

If a lesbian couple want a biological child (and they are not using a surrogate mother), they must decide who will carry the baby. "There are couples where one woman has always wanted to carry a child and the other one would rather eat rocks than be pregnant," says Drucker. At first, neither Angela nor Jackie wanted to get pregnant. Angela says, "Probably since I was 20, I knew I wanted children, but I knew I didn't want to have them physically." She concedes, "I would have, but something switched with Jackie and I was very grateful for it. One day she woke up and the biological clock struck 12, and she decided that she actually wanted to have a baby. And that worked out for me because I really didn't want to."

Jackie, who was trained as a therapist, decided to stay at home and raise their son. "I belong to a moms' club now, and I brought Adam to Mommy and Me class. I tell everybody [that I'm a lesbian]. I don't hide it. And some people do shy away and are not receptive, but, generally, most people are accepting. I also don't live in the middle of Wisconsin."

Jason and Tim are the parents of 17-month-old Noah. The two fathers say that because they live in a big city – Los Angeles – not many people are shocked by their family. However, they are asked the "Where's Mommy?" question. Jason, a film writer, observes, "People will notice a man alone with a baby more often than they will notice a woman alone with a baby. So we get asked a lot 'Where's Mommy?' And I don't know that a woman with a child, or two women with a child, would get asked 'Where's Daddy?' People expect to see a woman and a baby. So a man and a baby, or both of us and a baby, I think they notice us more." But Jason says that being a parent has "really opened the door for other people to feel like they can relate to us, people who might otherwise feel weird about the gay thing."

Even though society is now more tolerant of families headed by same-sex parents, gay and lesbian parents still face criticism. Opponents of same-sex parenting claim that gays and lesbians are raising children who will themselves become homosexuals, and that children need a mother and a father, not two of one. To the extent that that even matters, research indicates that children of gay and lesbian parents are no more likely to be homosexual than are children of heterosexual parents.[128]

Many same-sex parents actively seek out role models of the opposite sex for their children. The role model can be a friend of the couple's, a teacher, a relative, or a member of the clergy. Angela talks about the male role models her son, Adam, has in his life, including a 60-year-old neighbor across the street. "Adam just likes to go over there and sit on his knee. His name is Miles, and Miles gives him licorice. So that's a male figure. And we also have friends, Tom and Mark, who are male role models. ... I have two brothers and nephews and cousins. He sees them only a few times a year, but he still has fun hanging out with them," she notes.

Jason and Tim say little Noah has plenty of female role models in his life: his grandmothers and nanny, as well as Jason's best friend. Tim notes, "I'm not sure that there's any specific reason we want him [to be exposed to female role models], except that at a gut level, I know it's important, if for no other reason, than for him to have some experience with that before going to school and dealing with it."

Now that Noah is getting older, Jason and Tim want to make sure he understands that it is acceptable to have a family with two fathers. "We do this now in stories. We point to pictures and say that some families have only one mommy and then a daddy who lives somewhere else. And some families have a grandma and a grandpa. Some families have a daddy and a papa," explains Tim. Noah has a daddy, Jason, and a papa, Tim.

No matter which path to parenthood people take, they usually arrive at the same place. They experience many of the same joys and disappointments, as their lives are forever transformed. Jackie remarks, "Everything I do has changed. I'm no longer focused on myself. I'm focused on my family and my child, and I like it. I never thought I'd be that person, for whom driving a station wagon would be OK."

Conclusion

The journey to parenthood begins long before the baby arrives, long before expectant parents ever set eyes on the new life they have created. As young children, we start to take a mental inventory of our interactions with our parents, noting what has made us feel happy, safe and secure, and what has made us feel sad, mad and disappointed. These observations help us define what type of parent we would like to become.

There is no one psychological pathway to parenthood. Every couple's experience is shaped by a unique set of circumstances: childhood memories of their own parents, their observations of other parents – both in real life and in the media – and by the type of relationship they have with each other. The extent to which they buy into cultural definitions of parental roles also affects their journeys. In other words, it is personal experiences, shared experiences as a couple, and popular perceptions about motherhood and fatherhood, that together chart the way.

We tend to spend a great deal of time focusing on some of the more superficial trappings of new babyhood – obsessing over the perfect bedding for the crib and pre-enrolling babies in the "right" Mommy & Me classes before they are even born – and little or no time considering how this transition will change our lives. The goal of this book is to help people to begin preparing for their new roles well in advance of delivery so that the transition is an easier one. Expectant parents should try to imagine what life will be like after the baby arrives, not just a fairytale version, but a realistic one in which personal time, couple time, sleep time and patience may all be in short supply. LeeRan describes, "It's great, but it's hard. It's rewarding, but it's tough."

Expectant couples need to plan and prepare, not to guarantee a result, but to open their minds to the enormity of the life changes they are about to experience so that they will be better equipped to cope with what may come their way. The pregnancy period is an opportunity to run through a psychological dress rehearsal of what life may be like after the baby is born. It is unrealistic to think that expectant parents can strategize for every conceivable scenario related to new parenthood. However, they can use the nine months of pregnancy to begin to reflect on how a baby will affect their relationship, their individual identities and their day-to-day lives. They may also find it helpful to discuss what expectations they have of themselves and of their partner.

Pregnancy is also a good time for expectant parents to start to determine what kind of division of labor they would like to put in place for the postpartum period (and beyond) in order to take care of the burgeoning household and childcare responsibilities. In addition, they should mobilize their resources by arranging for some form of assistance – a doula, baby nurse, housekeeper, family member or friend – to help with the enormous postpartum workload. Having an extra set of hands can go a long way in reducing anxiety and allowing new parents to catch up on some much-needed sleep.

Finally, expectant and new parents should be aware that the realities of parenthood may not match their expectations. This is quite common. After all, how can expectant parents possibly know what it feels like to be responsible for the survival and emotional well-being of their own child until the baby arrives? As parents, we learn as we go. And we keep going as we learn.

Exploration questions

Pregnancy is a time of transformation. Give yourself permission to acknowledge all your feelings, regardless of what they may be. There are no right or wrong feelings. They speak the truth about your experience. Taking the time to question and understand yourself better is critical to your emotional well-being in the postpartum period. This process of exploration can be a valuable part of your transition to parenthood.

Decisions and myths

1 Go back in your mind as far as you can to the time when you first knew that you wanted a child. How old were you? Do you remember where you were, what you were doing or whom you were with? How did you know that you wanted a child?
2 As a couple, when did you realize that you wanted children? Recall the discussion you had. Did one of you want children more than the other? How did you decide that you would go forward and have a child? You should each make a list of four reasons why you wanted to have a child.
3 Make a list of everything that excites you about having a baby.
4 Make a list of everything that worries you about having a baby. (For questions #3 and #4, make separate lists and then discuss them with each other.)
5 How do you see your life changing? What will be different? Be specific.
6 What are the beliefs or stereotypes (including those from the media) about motherhood *and* fatherhood that you grew up with? You should each make these lists. How are your lists similar? How are they different?
7 (For each of you.) What is your favorite television program that revolves around family life? Give three reasons why it is your favorite.
8 What skills do you imagine it takes to parent a child? Which of those skills do you believe you have?
9 What changes do you believe you need to make in order to become the kind of parent that you want to be?
10 Do you want a girl or a boy? Will the sex of your child make a difference to you? If so, why? What are your beliefs about girls and boys? What would it be like to raise a girl? What would it be like to raise a boy?

Physiological experiences and the mind–body connection of pregnancy

1 Think back to the moment you found out that you were pregnant. How did you find out (i.e. pregnancy test, missed period)? What was your reaction? What was your partner's reaction when you told him or her?

2 (Women) What were your feelings about your body before you got pregnant? What are your feelings now? Why do you feel this way?

3 (Men) How do you feel about your partner's changing body? What part of her body do you find most appealing? What part of her body do you wish looked different?

4 What was it like the first time you saw your baby on the ultrasound?

5 What do you remember about the first time you felt your baby kick or move? Where were you? What were you doing? What do you remember feeling?

6 Do either of you have any fears or anxieties about procedures you will be undergoing as part of the prenatal care (i.e. blood tests, amniocentesis)? If so, make a list of what they are so that you can discuss them with your obstetrician or midwife. If you have already undergone a certain procedure, what was it like? Did it have an impact on your connection with your unborn child?

7 If you had a miscarriage before this pregnancy, talk with each other about any anxieties you may have about the possibility of losing the child you're pregnant with now. Because of that previous loss, do you worry that you will not be able to form a relationship with this child who is growing inside you?

8 (Women) Make a list of the changes you see in your body. What other changes do you expect to see as the pregnancy progresses?
(Men) Make a list of the changes you see in your partner's body. What other changes do you expect to see as the pregnancy progresses?

9 (Women) Have your ideas about your sexuality changed since you found out that you were pregnant? How so?
(Men) As you look at your partner's growing belly, how have your feelings about her as a sexual partner changed? Are you aware of any fears that either of you may have about making love during this time? Talk about other ways the two of you can express your affection for each other as the pregnancy progresses and sex becomes more cumbersome.

10 (Women) Write down the ways you will nourish your body and your baby during this pregnancy. What foods will you eat? What kinds of exercise will you do? Will you engage in bodywork like yoga to help you feel more connected to your changing body?

Mothers-to-be

1 List three qualities that make a "good mother." How did you learn this?

2 Are you having any mixed feelings about this pregnancy or about motherhood? If so, how long have you been having these feelings? What is your ambivalence about? Is it intensifying or diminishing as your pregnancy progresses?

3 Do you believe that you need to make any changes within yourself in order to be a good parent? If so, what changes do you need to make? Do you believe that you have the three "good mother" qualities you listed in your answer to Question 1?

4 Make a list of your mother's good parental qualities. List the things she did that you hope to repeat with your own children.

5 Make a list of the needs that you feel weren't met by your mother, and the things that you wish could have been different. For example, "I wish my mother had been more affectionate," or "I don't remember ever going shopping or out to lunch with my mother."

6 What is your current relationship with your mother and father? Has your relationship changed since you became pregnant? If your parents are deceased, are there any issues you had with them that remain unresolved in your mind?

7 Write down the kind of relationship you would like to have with your mother after you give birth. Is this relationship different from the one you have now? What kind of relationship do you think you'll actually have? How involved do you want your mother to be in your life?

8 Make a timeline of your relationship with your mother, starting with the very first memory that comes to mind. Then continue to remember your life with your mother, including both positive events (at least two) and negative events (at least two) that occurred in your relationship. (Sometimes looking at photographs of yourself with your mother can help you remember your life with her.)

9 Now visualize the kind of relationship that you want to have with your own child. What kinds of things do you imagine doing together?

10 What is your current work situation? What is your schedule like? Will you have the same schedule once you return to work after the baby is born? Does your employer offer flex-time, telecommuting or job sharing? How do you feel about balancing your new role as a mom with your role as a professional?

11 If you are planning to stop working, what feelings do you have about being with your child at home? Did your own mother stay at home or did she work outside the home? What did that mean in your life as a little girl? For example, did you come home from school by yourself? If your mother worked, was she able to come to school events and activities? What do you remember?

Fathers-to-be

1 Was this a planned or unplanned pregnancy? Do you remember your reaction when you found out about it?

2 How do you think that having a baby will affect your lifestyle? If you don't believe that it will affect it, are there specific reasons for this?

3 What kind of father do you want to be? Do you have to make any changes in order to become that kind of father?

4 Make a list of your father's good parental qualities. List the things he did that you hope to repeat with your own children.

5 Make a list of the needs that you feel weren't met by your father and the things that you wish could have been different. For example, "I wish my father had spent more time with me," or "I wish my father had taken me to a basketball game."

6 Visualize yourself as a father. What images come to mind?

7 As you imagine yourself in this new role of father, what kinds of fears come to mind?

8 Write down your definition of a "good father." How did you learn this?

9 Are you having any ambivalent feelings about this pregnancy? If so, what kinds of conflicting feelings have you been having? Are your feelings intensifying or diminishing as you near the end of this pregnancy?

10 Are any of your feelings about impending fatherhood related to your experiences with your own dad?

11 Make a list of the things that you missed having in your relationship with your father. Perhaps you wish that the two of you had spent more time together, or that he had talked with you more. Maybe you wish he had told you how much he loved you, or showed you more affection. Creating a list will help you to lay the foundation for your own identity as a father.

12 How has your mother influenced your feelings about the kind of father you want to be? How has this affected your expectations about the kind of mothering you want for your child?

Labor and delivery

1 Where do you want to give birth (i.e. at home, in the hospital, at a birthing center)?

2 Is there anyone else, besides the two of you, whom you want to be present at the birth of your child?

3 What kind of environment do you want to create for yourself if you deliver away from home? What special things would you like to have with you to create a feeling of home and the familiar (i.e. a special blanket or pillow, a favorite kind of music that you find relaxing)?

4 Will you have a doula/midwife in the delivery room as a labor coach? Why did you want to have a doula/midwife assist you?

5 (Men) What will be your role during labor and delivery? If your partner has an unexpected cesarean section, do you want to be present? If not, why? Are you afraid of blood or worried that you will faint? Make a list of your fears so that you can address them with your healthcare provider, and then arrange things in such a way that you will be comfortable attending the birth of your child.

6 (Women) What will be your partner's role? What do you imagine you will need from him?

7 (Women) Who will make decisions for you in the event that you are unable to make them for yourself?

8 (Men and women) Make a list of the things that worry you about labor and delivery. You should discuss these concerns with your physician, midwife, doula or nurse practitioner.

9 (Women) Write down your feelings about your visits to the doctor/midwife, including how you feel about your relationship with him or her. Are there things that you want to talk about that embarrass you? Do you feel that your healthcare provider takes your concerns seriously?

10 Think about whether or not you want to have a birth plan. What kinds of things would you include in this plan? If you do create one, write it during the second trimester so that you have time to discuss it with your doctor and modify it, if necessary, well in advance of delivery.

11 Make a list of the advantages of having a birth plan.

12 What do you know about yourself and how you respond in situations where things don't turn out the way you had anticipated?

13 (Women) Is there anything in your past that you believe could affect your experience of childbirth? For example, were you molested, or is there some shame that you feel about your body?

Welcoming baby

1 What images do you have of your new baby arriving home? Close your eyes and visualize how it will feel to hold your baby in your arms as you walk through the front door. What feelings are awakened by these images (i.e. joy, fear, anxiety, elation)? Talk with each other about what feelings surface and why you think you might be feeling that way.

2 Imagine what it would be like to spend a day with your baby.

3 If you have not already done so, make a specific plan about what support system you will have for the first two months. Write down the names and phone numbers of everyone who might be able to help you after the baby comes home.

• **Keep in mind:** Aside from immediate family, other people – close friends, neighbors and co-workers – can provide assistance during the postpartum period. Additionally, paid professionals, such as baby nurses, doulas and housekeepers can help in reducing the tremendous postpartum workload. If you are a single parent, creating a support network is critical. Just remember that support is not only about physical assistance with housework and errands. New parents also need emotional support in the form of affection and encouragement.

- **Keep in mind:** Make a checklist now so that someone (a friend, relative or neighbor) will stock your refrigerator and freezer with nutritious foods that do not require any preparation (i.e. sliced meats, chopped vegetables and fruit, yogurt, hard-boiled eggs, sliced cheese, bottled water and juice).

4 Think honestly about how you have handled major changes in the past. Do you associate change with adventure or disaster? As you reflect on previous experiences, which of them have generally made you the most anxious? How did you cope? Were your coping methods helpful?

5 In the past, how have you handled disappointment? Within a couple of weeks postpartum, make a list of some of the things that disappointed you about your labor and delivery. For example, maybe you were disappointed with your baby's gender or his appearance. This is a task for both new moms and dads. Perhaps you had a cesarean section when you desperately wanted a vaginal, drug-free delivery. Maybe breastfeeding is not proceeding as you had anticipated. Go into as much detail as possible. In some cases, you may want to contact a therapist who is knowledgeable about postpartum issues to help you process your childbirth experience.

- **Keep in mind:** Talk with each other about how you want to handle the flow of visitors. Perhaps you want to record an outgoing message on your answering machine letting callers know that you have just had a baby and may not be able to return calls or accept visitors for a few days.

6 (For expectant parents with family living out of town.) Who will be coming and when? Will they just be visiting, or will they also be helping? Do they know whether they are expected to help? Will they be staying in your house overnight or at a hotel? Are you concerned about intrusive family members?

- **Keep in mind:** Think about how you can stagger visitors. It is especially helpful to decide this in advance so that each of you can communicate your decision to your own parents, as well as other relatives and friends. Talk now about some of the boundaries that you want to establish. The most important thing for a new mother is to feel competent. And a meddling mother or mother-in-law can sometimes make a new mom feel inadequate and anxious.

- **Keep in mind:** The early weeks postpartum should be a time when the new mother is recovering from childbirth and the last-trimester challenges of her pregnancy. Sleep is critical. Others can help her recuperate by preparing meals, handling the grocery shopping and other errands, writing thank-you notes, and doing the dishes or the laundry.

The changing marital relationship

1 Make your own lists of how you see your relationship changing (i.e. less physical intimacy, less time spent with each other). Then discuss any concerns you may have.

2 (Women) Make a list of the special qualities your partner has which you believe will make him a wonderful father, and then read it to him.
(Men) Write down the special qualities that your partner has which you believe will make her a wonderful mother, and then read it to her.

3 (Men) Visualize your partner becoming the mother of your child. Will you have trouble continuing to view her as a sexual being? Explain your answer.
(Women) As you look ahead to becoming a mother, how do you imagine your sense of self, your sense of femininity and the way you view yourself as a sexual being will change?

4 Talk about how you can honor your relationship after the baby is born.

5 (Women) How do you expect your partner will help with baby care and household chores?

6 (Men) How would you like to be able to participate in baby care and other domestic responsibilities?

7 (Men) Think back to your childhood family and your relationship with your own siblings. If you were the oldest, think about how you felt when your brother or sister was born. Did you feel less important? Did you ever feel as if you had to compete for attention?

Postpartum depression

1 Have any of your female relatives (mother, grandmother, sisters, aunts) ever experienced depression during pregnancy or in the postpartum period?

2 Does anyone in your family (either male or female) have a history of bipolar disorder or schizophrenia?

3 Have you or any close female relatives experienced hormonally related difficulties, such as premenstrual dysphoric disorder (PMDD)?

4 Are you currently taking any medications (prescription or over-the-counter) on a regular basis?

5 Have you ever been treated for depression, anxiety or other mood-related disorders? Were you treated with medication and/or therapy? Have you or any of your relatives experienced mood changes that lasted for more than two weeks?

6 Did you have any childhood experiences of physical or sexual abuse, emotional abuse or neglect?

7 Have you or any of your relatives been treated for substance abuse?

8 Have you ever had a miscarriage or a stillbirth? Have you ever terminated a pregnancy?

- **Keep in mind:** Because pregnancy is such a powerful physiological and psychological experience, the painful memories of previous losses, such as a parent's death, or a miscarriage, may resurface. And this can put a woman at a greater risk of developing depression after childbirth.

9 During this pregnancy, are you experiencing any major life stressors (e.g. moving to a new house, a change or loss of job, financial difficulties)?

- **Keep in mind:** Some stresses are unavoidable. It is important to take an inventory of the stressors in your life and to discuss ways that you can reduce the impact on your body (i.e. enlisting additional help with a move, talking to a therapist in order to cope with the loss of a loved one). Make a list of coping resources that you could use.

- **Keep in mind:** If you answered "yes" to any of the above questions, particularly those concerning a personal or family history of depression or anxiety, it is crucial to let your obstetrician, midwife, doula and/or internist know that you fall into one of the risk categories for postpartum depression so that a support plan can be implemented during pregnancy.

The many paths to parenthood

Adoption

1 Why did you decide to adopt a child?
2 What kind of adoption did you choose and why? Open or closed? Domestic or international? An agency adoption or an independent adoption?
3 What are the age and gender of the child you would like to adopt?
4 If you are considering an open adoption, what kind of relationship do you envision having with the birth mother during pregnancy and after delivery?
5 As a couple, do the two of you feel differently about adopting? If so, explain why you feel differently.
6 If you are planning to adopt because of infertility issues, what feelings are connected with your decision?

Infertility

1 Have you had any miscarriages, stillbirths or abortions? If so, how many?
2 If you have experienced a pregnancy loss, do you feel that you have mourned that loss? If not, what has hindered this?
3 What options are you exploring (i.e. IVF, GIFT, sperm or egg donation, surrogacy)?
4 Are you prepared to cope with the possibility of a multiple birth?
5 Talk with each other about how your fertility issues have affected your relationship. Has it changed the way you view intimacy?

Single moms

These questions are geared toward women who are single mothers by choice.

1 Why did you decide to become a single mother? What experiences in your life led you to this decision?
2 How are you planning to have a child? By getting pregnant? Adopting?
3 How do you plan to get pregnant? By using a sperm donor or by having sexual intercourse with a man you know? Will he be involved in parenting the child?
4 Make a list of the advantages and disadvantages of raising a child alone.
5 What emotions surface when you complete your list? Are there any feelings of sadness or loss that emerge when you think about raising this child alone? What are some of the ways you can address these feelings?
6 Make a list of all the people who might be part of your support team. Write down the names of everyone you can think of, regardless of whether you know how they can provide support.

Stay-at-home dads

1 (Men) What were the factors that influenced your decision (i.e. economics, personality type, individual career goals)?
2 What might be some of the advantages for your family of reversing the traditional roles? Disadvantages?
3 (Men) Do you worry about the reaction of family, friends or other people? If so, what are your concerns?
4 (Men) Will you also work part-time?
5 (Men) What kinds of responsibilities will you have as a stay-at-home dad?

- **Keep in mind:** Joining a support organization and talking to other families with stay-at-home dads can be helpful.

Same-sex parents

1 If you are a gay couple, will you adopt? Do you want to adopt an infant or an older child?
2 If you are a lesbian couple and you decide on pregnancy, who will carry the baby? What factors helped you reach this decision? If you are planning to have more than one child, is it important to you that they are biologically related?
3 In your particular state, what are the laws regarding same-sex couples and adoption?
4 What kinds of roles and responsibilities will each person have?
5 Will you both continue to work? If so, how does this affect your thinking about your roles at home?

References

1 LeMasters EE. Parenthood as crisis. *Marriage Fam Liv.* 1957; **21:** 251–5.

2 Dyer ED. Parenthood as crisis: a re-study. *Marriage Fam Liv.* 1963; **25:** 196–201.

3 Hobbs DF. Parenthood as crisis: a third study. *J Marriage Fam.* 1965; **27:** 367–89.

4 Cowan CP, Cowan PA. *When Partners Become Parents: the big life change for couples.* Mahwah, NJ: Lawrence Erlbaum Associates, Inc; 1992.

5 Belsky J, Pensky E. Marital change across the transition to parenthood. *Marriage Fam Rev.* 1988; **12:** 133–56.

6 Cowan CP, Cowan PA. *When Partners Become Parents: the big life change for couples.* Mahwah, NJ: Lawrence Erlbaum Associates; 1992.

7 Belsky J, Spanier GB, Rovine M. Stability and change in marriage across the transition to parenthood. *J Marriage Fam.* 1983; **45:** 567–77.

8 Draper J. It was a real good show: the ultrasound scan, fathers and the power of visual knowledge. *Soc Health Illness.* 2002; **24:** 771–95.

9 Wirth F. *Prenatal Parenting: the complete psychological and spiritual guide to loving your unborn child.* New York: Harper Collins; 2001.

10 Affonso DD, Mayberry LJ. Common stressors reported by a group of childbearing American women. *Health Care Women Int.* 1990; **11:** 331–45.

11 American College of Obstetricians and Gynecologists. *You and Your Baby.* Pamphlet. Washington, D.C.: American College of Obstetricians and Gynecologists; 1999.

12 Conner GK, Denson V. Expectant fathers' response to pregnancy: review of literature and implications for research in high-risk pregnancy. *J Perinat Neonat Nurs.* 1990; **4:** 33–42.

13 Masoni S, Maio A, Trimarchi G *et al.* The couvade syndrome. *J Psychosom Obstet Gynaecol.* 1994; **15:** 125–31.

14 Bogren LY. Changes in sexuality in women and men during pregnancy. *Arch Sex Behav.* 1991; **20:** 35–45.

15 Sayle A, Savitz DA, Thorp JM *et al.* Sexual activity during late pregnancy and risk of preterm delivery. *Obstet Gynaecol.* 2001; **97:** 283–9.

16 Janov A. *The Biology of Love.* New York: Prometheus Publishing; 2000.

17 Martin JA, Hamilton BE, Sutton PD *et al.* Births: final data for 2003. *Natl Vital Stat Rep.* 2005; **54:** 1–116.

18 Martin JA, Hamilton BE, Sutton PD *et al.* Births: final data for 2002. *Natl Vital Stat Rep.* 2003; **52:** 1–114.

19 Martin JA, Hamilton BE, Sutton PD *et al.* Births: final data for 2001. *Natl Vital Stat Rep.* 2002; **51**: 1–103.

20 Lerner H. *The Mother Dance: how children change your life.* New York: Harper Collins Publishers; 1998.

21 Glade AC, Bean RA, Vera R. A prime time for marital/relational intervention: a review of the transition to parenthood literature with treatment recommendations. *Am J Fam Therapy.* 2005; **33**: 319–36.

22 Secunda V. *Women and Their Fathers: the sexual and romantic impact of the first man in your life.* New York: Delacorte Press; 1992.

23 Edelman H. *Motherless Daughters: the legacy of loss.* Reading, MA: Addison-Wesley Publishing; 1994.

24 Shereshefsky PM, Yarrow LJ. *Psychological Aspects of a First Pregnancy and Early Postnatal Adaptation.* New York: Raven Press; 1973.

25 ABC Poll, *ABC News Good Morning America*/Good Housekeeping Poll. Data collection by TNS of Horsham, PA, April 2006.

26 Hays S. *The Cultural Contradictions of Motherhood.* New Haven, CT: Yale University Press; 1996.

27 Winnicott DW. *Babies and Their Mothers.* London: Free Association Books; 1987.

28 Warner J. *Perfect Madness: motherhood in the age of anxiety.* New York: Riverhead Books; 2005.

29 U.S. Census Bureau. *Current Population Survey, March and Annual Social and Economic Supplements,* 2005 and earlier. Washington, D.C.: U.S. Census Bureau; 2006.

30 Dye JL. *Fertility of American Women. Current population reports.* Washington, D.C.: U.S. Census Bureau; 2004.

31 Downs B. *Fertility of American Women: June 2002. Current population reports.* Washington, D.C.: U.S. Census Bureau; 2003.

32 U.S. Census Bureau. *Employment Characteristics of Families in 2004. Current population survey.* Washington, D.C.: Bureau of Labor Statistics, U.S. Census Bureau; 2005.

33 Lupton D, Barclay L. *Constructing Fatherhood: discourses and experiences.* Thousand Oaks, CA: Sage Publications; 1997.

34 Shapiro JL. *The Measure of a Man: becoming the man you wish your father had been.* New York: Delacorte Press; 1993.

35 Dooley C, Fedele N. *Mothers and Sons: raising relational boys.* Wellesley, MA: Wellesley Centers for Women, Wellesley College; 1999.

36 Gurian M. *Mothers, Sons and Lovers: how a man's relationship with his mother affects the rest of his life.* Boston, MA: Shambhala Publications; 1994.

37 Bond JT, Thompson CT, Galinsky E *et al. Highlights of the National Study of the Changing Workforce.* New York: Families and Work Institute; 2003.

38 Families and Work Institute. *Generation and Gender in the Workplace Study.* New York: Families and Work Institute, The American Business Collaboration; 2004.

39 Bond JT, Thompson CT, Galinsky E et al. Highlights of the National Study of the Changing Workforce. New York: Families and Work Institute; 2003.

40 Lino M. Expenditures on children by families, 2005. Miscellaneous Publication Number 1528–2005. Alexandria, VA: USDA Center for Nutrition Policy and Promotion; 2006.

41 Duvall EM. Family Development. 4th ed. New York: J.B. Lippincott Company; 1971.

42 Glazer G. Anxiety and stressors of expectant fathers. West J Nurs Res. 1989; **11:** 47–59.

43 Affonso DD, Mayberry LJ. Common stressors reported by a group of childbearing American woman. Health Care Women Int. 1990; **11:** 331–45.

44 Dip G, Hopper U, Moorem M. Do birth plans empower women? Evaluation of a hospital birth plan. Birth. 1995; **22:** 29–36.

45 Whitford HM, Hillian EM. Women's perceptions of birth plans. Midwifery. 1998; **14:** 248–53.

46 Shapiro JL. The Measure of a Man: becoming the man you wish your father had been. New York: Delacorte Press; 1993.

47 Declercq ED, Sakala C, Corry MP et al. Listening to Mothers. II. Report of the Second National U.S. Survey of Women's Childbearing Experiences. New York: Childbirth Connection; 2006.

48 Leavitt JW. Brought to Bed: Child-bearing in America, 1750–1950. New York: Oxford University Press; 1986.

49 Vehvilainen-Julkunen K, Liukkonen A. Fathers' experiences of childbirth. Midwifery. 1998; **14:** 10–17.

50 Chan KK, Paterson-Brown S. How do fathers feel accompanying their partners in labor and delivery? J Obstet Gynaecol. 2002; **22:** 11–15.

51 Wuitchik M, Hesson K, Bakal DA. Perinatal predictors of pain and distress during labor. Birth. 1990; **17:** 186–91.

52 Declercq ED, Sakala C, Corry MP et al. Listening to Mothers. II. Report of the Second National U.S. Survey of Women's Childbearing Experiences. New York: Childbirth Connection; 2006.

53 Martin JA, Hamilton BE, Sutton PD et al. Births: final data for 2003. Natl Vital Stat Rep. 2005; **54:** 1–116.

54 Government Statistical Service for the Department of Health. NHS Maternity Statistics. England: 2003–04. London: Department of Health; 2005.

55 Martin JA, Hamilton BE, Sutton PD et al. Births: final data for 2003. Natl Vital Stat Rep. 2005; **54:** 1–116.

56 Linden DW, Paroli ET, Doron MW. Preemies: the essential guide for parents of premature babies. New York: Pocket Books; 2000.

57 Linden DW, Paroli ET, Doron MW. Preemies: the essential guide for parents of premature babies. New York: Pocket Books; 2000.

58 Hoyert DL, Heron MP, Murphy SL *et al.* Deaths: final data for 2003. *Natl Vital Stat Rep.* 2006; **54:** 1–120.

59 Richardson H. Kangaroo care: why does it work? *Midwifery Today.* 1997; **44:** 50–1.

60 Charpak N, Ruiz-Peláez, JG, Figueroa de CZ *et al.* Kangaroo mother versus traditional care for newborn infants ≤ 2000 grams: a randomized, controlled trial. *Pediatrics.* 1997; **100:** 682–8.

61 Gale G, VandenBerg KA. Developmental care. *Neonatal Network.* 1998; **17:** 69–71.

62 Hoyert DL, Heron MP, Murphy SL *et al.* Deaths: final data for 2003. *Natl Vital Stat Rep.* 2006; **54:** 1–120.

63 American Academy of Pediatrics. The changing concept of sudden infant death syndrome: diagnostic coding shifts, controversies regarding the sleep environment, and new variables to consider in reducing risk. *Pediatrics.* 2005; **116:** 1245–55.

64 Lee E, Furedi F. *Mothers' Experience of and Attitudes to Using Infant Formula in the Early Months.* Canterbury: School of Social Policy, Sociology and Social Research, University of Kent; 2005.

65 Centers for Disease Control and Prevention. *National Immunization Survey, 2005.* Atlanta, GA: Centers for Disease Control and Prevention, Department of Health and Human Services; 2006; www.cdc.gov/breastfeeding/data/NIS data/data 2005.htm

66 Allen SM, Hawkins AJ. Maternal gatekeeping: mothers' beliefs and behaviors that inhibit greater father involvement in family work. *J Marriage Fam.* 1999; **61:** 199–212.

67 Belsky J, Pensky E. Marital change across the transition to parenthood. *Marriage Fam Rev.* 1988; **12:** 133–56.

68 Cowan CP, Cowan PA. *When Partners Become Parents: the big life change for couples.* Mahwah, NJ: Lawrence Erlbaum Associates; 1992.

69 Belsky J, Spanier GB, Rovine M. Stability and change in marriage across the transition to parenthood. *J Marriage Fam.* 1983; **45:** 567–77.

70 Hobbs DF. Parenthood as crisis: a third study. *J Marriage Fam.* 1965; **27:** 367–72.

71 Dyer ED. Parenthood as crisis: a re-study. *Marriage Fam Liv.* 1963; **25:** 196–201.

72 LeMasters EE. Parenthood as crisis. *Marriage Fam Liv.* 1957; **21:** 251–5.

73 Winnicott DW. *Collected Papers: through paediatrics to psycho-analysis.* London: Tavistock Publications; 1958.

74 Belsky J, Pensky E. Marital change across the transition to parenthood. *Marriage Fam Rev.* 1988; **12:** 133–56.

75 Cowan CP, Cowan PA. *When Partners Become Parents: the big life change for couples.* Mahwah, NJ: Lawrence Erlbaum Associates; 1992.

76 Belsky J, Spanier GB, Rovine M. Stability and change in marriage across the transition to parenthood. *J Marriage Fam.* 1983; **45:** 567–77.

77 Shapiro AF, Gottman JM, Carrer S. The baby and the marriage: identifying factors that buffer against decline in marital satisfaction after the first baby arrives. *J Fam Psychiatry.* 2000; **14:** 59–70.

78 Delmore-Ko P, Pancer MS, Hunsberger B *et al.* Becoming a parent: the relation between prenatal expectations and postnatal experience. *J Fam Psychiatry.* 2000; **14:** 625–40.

79 Cowan CP, Cowan PA, Heming G *et al.* Transitions to parenthood: his, hers and theirs. *J Fam Issues.* 1985; **6:** 451–81.

80 Levy-Shiff R. Individual and contextual correlates of marital change across the transition to parenthood. *Dev Psychol.* 1994; **30:** 591–601.

81 Belsky J, Spanier GB, Rovine M. Stability and change in marriage across the transition to parenthood. *J Marriage Fam.* 1983; **45:** 567–77.

82 Belsky J, Lang ME, Rovine M. Stability and change in marriage across the transition to parenthood: a second study. *J Marriage Fam.* 1985; **47:** 855–65.

83 Gottman JM, Silver N. *The Seven Principles for Making Marriage Work.* New York: Three Rivers Press; 1999.

84 Hyde JS, Delamater JD, Plant EA *et al.* Sexuality during pregnancy and the year postpartum. *J Sex Res.* 1996; **33:** 143–51.

85 Janov A. *The Biology of Love.* New York: Prometheus Publishing; 2000.

86 Hyde JS, Delamater JD, Plant EA *et al.* Sexuality during pregnancy and the year postpartum. *J Sex Res.* 1996; **33:** 143–51.

87 American Psychiatric Association. *Diagnostic and Statistical Manual of Mental Disorders.* 4th ed. Washington, D.C.: American Psychiatric Association; 1994.

88 Robins LN, Regier DA, editors. *Psychiatric Disorders in America: the epidemiologic catchment area study.* New York: The Free Press; 1990.

89 O'Hara MW, Swain AM. Rates and risks of postpartum depression: a meta-analysis. *Int Rev Psychiatry.* 1996; **8:** 37–54.

90 Ramchandani P, Stein A, Evans J *et al.* Paternal depression in the postnatal period and child development: a prospective population study. *Obstet Gynecol Surv.* 2005; **60:** 789–90.

91 Burke L. The impact of maternal depression on familial relationships. *Int Rev Psychiatry.* 2003; **15:** 243–55.

92 Beck CT. The effects of postpartum depression on maternal–infant interaction: a meta-analysis. *Nurs Res.* 1995; **44:** 298–304.

93 Goodman JH. Paternal postpartum depression, its relationship to maternal postpartum depression, and implications for family health. *J Adv Nurs.* 2004; **45:** 26–35.

94 American Thyroid Association. *Patient Education Overview. Postpartum thyroiditis FAQ.* Falls Church, VA: American Thyroid Assosciation; 2004.

95 Gotlib IH, Whiffen VE, Mount JH *et al.* Prevalence rates and demographic characteristics associated with depression in pregnancy and the postpartum. *J Consult Clin Psychol.* 1989; **57:** 269–74.

96 Levine RE, Oandasan AP, Primeau LA *et al.* Anxiety disorders during pregnancy and postpartum. *Am J Perinatol.* 2003; **20**: 239–48.

97 Andersson L, Sundstrom-Poromaa I, Bixo M *et al.* Point prevalence of psychiatric disorders during the second trimester of pregnancy: a population-based study. *Am J Obstet Gynecol.* 2003; **189**: 148–54.

98 Heron J, O'Connor TG, Evans J *et al.* The course of anxiety and depression through pregnancy and the postpartum in a community sample. *J Affect Disord.* 2004; **80**: 65–73.

99 Wadhwa PD. Psychoneuroendocrine processes in human pregnancy, influences in fetal development and health. *Psychoneuroendocrinology.* 2005; **30**: 724–43.

100 Sichel D, Driscoll JW. *Women's Moods: what every woman must know about hormones, the brain, and emotional health.* New York: Harper Collins; 1999.

101 Misri SK. *Pregnancy Blues: what every woman needs to know about depression during pregnancy.* New York: Delacorte Press; 2005.

102 Beck CT. Predictors of postpartum depression: an update. *Nurs Res.* 2001; **50**: 275–85.

103 Misri S, Kostaras X, Fox D *et al.* The impact of partner support in the treatment of postpartum depression. *Can J Psychiatry.* 2000; **45**: 554–8.

104 Boyce P, Hickey A. Psychosocial risk factors for major depression after childbirth. *Soc Psychiatry Psychiatr Epidemiol.* 2005; **40**: 605–12.

105 Cohen LS, Altshuler LL, Harlow BL *et al.* Relapse of major depression during pregnancy in women who maintain or discontinue antidepressant treatment. *JAMA.* 2006; **295**: 499–503.

106 O'Connor TG, Heron J, Glover V. Antenatal anxiety predicts child behavioural/emotional problems independently of postnatal depression. *J Am Acad Child and Adolescent Psych.* 2002; **41**(12): 1470–7.

107 Cooper PJ, Murray L. Postnatal depression. *BMJ.* 1998; **316**: 1884–6.

108 GlaxoSmithKlein. Updated preliminary report on bupropion and other antidepressants, including paroxetine in pregnancy and the occurrence of cardiovascular and major congenital malformation. Study No. EPIP083. December 13, 2005. www.gsk.com/media/paroxetine_pregnancy.htm.

109 Kallen B, Olausson PO. Antidepressant drugs during pregnancy and infant congenital heart defect. *Reprod Toxicol.* 2006: **21**: 221–2.

110 US Food and Drug Administration. Advising of risk of birth defects with Paxil: agency requiring updated product labelling. *FDA News.* 2005; **December 8**: press release.

111 Chambers CD, Hernandez-Diaz S, Van Marter LJ *et al.* Selective serotonin reuptake inhibitors: risk of persistent pulmonary hypertension of the newborn. *NEJM.* 2006; **354**: 579–87.

112 Levinson-Castiel R. Antidepressants in pregnancy linked to newborn hangover. *Arch Pediatr Adolesc Med.* 2006: **160**: 173–6.

113 Hallberg P, Sjoblom V. The use of selective serotonin reuptake inhibitors during pregnancy and breast-feeding: a review and clinical aspects. *J Clin Psychopharmacol*. 2005; **25**: 59–73.

114 Nonacs R. *A Deeper Shade of Blue: a Woman's Guide to Recognizing and Treating Depression in her Childbearing Years*. New York: Simon & Schuster; 2006.

115 Misri S, Kostaras X. Benefits and risks to mother and infant of drug treatment for postnatal depression. *Drug Safety*. 2002; **25**(13): 903–11.

116 Misri S, Kostaras X. Benefits and risks to mother and infant of drug treatment for postnatal depression. *Drug Safety*. 2002; **25**(13): 903–11.

117 Hale TW. *Medications and Mothers' Milk*. 12th ed. Amarillo, TX: Hale Publishing, L.P.; 2006.

118 Briggs GG, Freeman RK, Yaffe SJ. *Drugs in Pregnancy and Lactation*. Philadelphia, PA: Lippincott, Williams and Wilkins; 2005.

119 National Adoption Information Clearinghouse. Latest US adoption statistics show increase in public agency adoptions while total numbers remain constant. *Children's Bureau Express*. 2004/2005; **5**: press release.

120 European Society for Human Reproduction and Embryology. *Three million babies born using assisted reproductive technologies*. Press release, 22nd Annual Conference of the European Society for Human Reproduction and Embryology, Prague, 21 June 2006.

121 European Society for Human Reproduction and Embryology. *Three million babies born using assisted reproductive technologies*. Press release, 22nd Annual Conference of the European Society for Human Reproduction and Embryology, Prague, 21 June 2006.

122 Martin JA, Hamilton BE, Sutton PD *et al*. Births: final data for 2003. *Natl Vital Stat Rep*. 2005; **54**: 1–116.

123 Martin JA, Hamilton BE, Sutton PD *et al*. Births: final data for 2003. *Natl Vital Stat Rep*. 2005; **54**: 1–116.

124 Hilling H. *The Man Who Would Be Dad*. Sterling, VA: Capital Books; 2002.

125 U.S. Census Bureau. Parents and children in stay-at-home parent family groups: 1994 to present. In: *Current Population Survey. March and Annual Social and Economic Supplements, 2005 and earlier*. Washington, D.C.: U.S. Census Bureau; 2006.

126 Drucker J. *Lesbian and Gay Families Speak Out: understanding the joys and challenges of diverse family life*. New York: Perseus Publishing; 2001.

127 Human Rights Campaign Foundation. *The Cost of Marriage Inequality to Children and Their Same-Sex Parents*. Washington, D.C.: Human Rights Campaign Foundation; 2004.

128 Patterson J. Family relationships of lesbians and gay men. *J Marriage Fam*. 2000; **62**: 1052–69.

Resources

Adoption

- *Adoption Today* Magazine
  Tel: (888) 924 6736
  www.adoptinfo.net

- Foli KJ, Thompson JR. *The Post Adoption Blues.* New York, St.Martin's Press; 2004.

- Adoptive Families of America
  Tel: (800) 372 3300 (24-hour helpline)

- www.adoption.com

- www.adoption.org

- www.adoptionuk.org (for the U.K.)

Birth plans

- Wagner M. *Creating Your Birth Plan: a definitive guide to a safe and empowering birth.* New York: Perigee Books; 2006.

- www.birthplan.com

- www.childbirth.org

Breastfeeding

- La Leche League International. *The Womanly Art of Breastfeeding.* Revised 7th ed. New York: Plume; 2004.

- www.breastfeeding.com

- www.lalecheleague.org

Fatherhood

- Brott A. *The Expectant Father: facts, tips and advice for dads to be.* 2nd ed. New York: Abbeville Publishing; 2001.

- Diamond MJ. *My Father Before Me: how fathers and sons influence each other throughout their lives.* New York: W.W. Norton; 2007.

- Goldman MJ. *The Joy of Fatherhood.* New York: Three Rivers Press; 2000.

- www.fatherhood.org

- www.fathersdirect.com

Infertility

- Swire-Falker E. *The Infertility Survival Guide.* New York: Riverhead Books; 2004.

- American Fertility Association; www.theafa.org

  American Society for Reproductive Medicine; www.asrm.org

- International Council on Infertility Information Dissemination; www.inciid.org

- National Infertility Association; www.resolve.org

Labor and delivery

- Leavitt JW. *Brought to Bed: child-bearing in America, 1750–1950.* New York: Oxford University Press; 1986.

- Simkin P. *The Birth Partner: everything you need to know to help a woman through childbirth.* 2nd ed. Boston, MA: Harvard Common Press; 2001.

- www.bradleybirth.com

- www.hypnobirthing.com

- www.hypnobirthing.co.uk

- www.lamaze.org

Marriage and the transition to parenthood

- Cowan CP, Cowan PA. *When Partners Become Parents: the big life change for couples.* New York: Basic Books; 2000.

- Gottman JM, Silver N. *The Seven Principles for Making Marriage Work.* New York: Three Rivers Press; 1999.

- Jordan PL, Stanley SM, Markman HJ. *Becoming Parents: how to strengthen your marriage as your family grows.* New York: Jossey-Bass; 1999.

Motherhood

- Matthias R. *51 Secrets of Motherhood (That Your Mother Never Told You).* Trenton, NJ: Franklin Mason Press; 2005.

- Stern D, Bruschweiler-Stern N. *The Birth of a Mother.* New York: Basic Books; 1998.

- Warner J. *Perfect Madness: motherhood in the age of anxiety.* New York: Riverhead Books; 2005.

- Wolf N. *Misconceptions: truths, lies and the unexpected journey of motherhood.* New York: Anchor Books; 2003.

- www.netmums.com

- www.babyzone.com

- www.ivillage.com

- www.mommytoo.com

- www.workingmother.com

Postpartum depression

- Hanzak E. *Eyes Without Sparkle. Understanding the journey of postpartum illness.* Oxford: Radcliffe Publishing; 2005.

- Kleiman K. *The Postpartum Husband. Practical solutions for living with postpartum depression.* Philadelphia, PA: Xlibris; 2000.

- Kleiman K. *What Am I Thinking? Having a baby after postpartum depression.* Philadelphia, PA: Xlibris; 2005.

- Misri SK. *Pregnancy Blues: what every woman needs to know about depression during pregnancy.* New York: Delacorte Press; 2005.

- Poulin S. *The Mother-to-Mother Postpartum Depression Support Book: real stories from women who lived through it and recovered.* New York: Berkley Publishing; 2006.

- Postpartum Support International; www.postpartum.net

- www.postpartumprogress.com

- www.marcesociety.com

- www.elainehanzak.co.uk

Pregnancy and birth

- Douglas A. *The Mother of All Pregnancy Books: the ultimate guide to conception, birth and everything in between.* New York: Wiley Publishing; 2002.

- www.babycenter.com

- www.babycentre.co.uk

- www.babyzone.com

- www.birthpsychology.com

- www.childbirthconnection.org

Premature births

- Ludington-Hoe SM, Golant SK. *Kangaroo Care: the best you can do to help your preterm infant.* New York: Bantam; 1993.

- www.bliss.org.uk

- www.preemies.org

Same-sex parenting

- Drucker J. *Lesbian and Gay Families Speak Out: understanding the joys and challenges of diverse family life.* New York: Perseus Publishing; 2001.

- Lev AI. *The Complete Lesbian and Gay Parenting Guide.* New York: The Berkley Publishing Group; 2004.

- American Civil Liberties Union Lesbian and Gay Rights Project
  Tel: (212) 944 9800
  www.aclu.org/lgbt/index.html

- COLAGE: Children of Lesbians and Gays Everywhere
  Tel: (415) 861 KIDS
  www.colage.org/

- Family Pride Coalition
  Tel: (202) 331 5015
  www.familypride.org/

- www.popluck.org

- www.prideparenting.com (for the U.K.)

Single mothers

- Mattes J. *Single Mothers by Choice: a guidebook for single women who are considering or have chosen motherhood.* New York: Three Rivers Press; 1997.

- www.singlemothers.org

- www.mattes.home.pipeline.com

Stay-at-home fathers

- Hilling H. *The Man Who Would Be Dad.* Sterling, VA: Capital Books; 2002.

- www.slowlane.com

Index

52585

146 Index

umbilical cord 50, 51, 52
University of Wisconsin study 85, 86
unmarried mothers *see* single mothers
unplanned pregnancy 7, 9
U.S. Census Bureau 37, 109, 110
U.S. Department of Agriculture 46
uterus shape 61

vacuum extraction 59, 63
vaginal bleeding 25, 61
vaginal dryness 86
ventilators 70
ventouse 59, 63
Verny, Dr. Thomas 17
visitors 3, 12, 73–6, 100–1, 120
visual impairment 61
visualization 31
vitamins 27
vomiting 18, 22, 24, 51

Wall Street Journal 96
Warner, Judith 35
water birth 59
websites 52, 65, 131–5
weight gain
  body image 1, 17, 18, 19–20, 21
  couvade syndrome 23, 24, 40
  premature babies 62
  sex after baby 85
welcoming baby home 65–76
  advice 75–6
  bonding 71–2

breastfeeding 66–7
caring for newest family
    member 65–6
exploration questions 119–21
maintaining perspective 68–71
new division of labor 72–3
overview 2, 65
postpartum game plan 76
visitors 73–5
Winnicott, D.W. 35, 79
Wirth, Frederick 17
withdrawal syndrome 98
Woman's Mental Health Program,
    Emory University 97
women's movement 46
work
  body image 18, 19, 20
  exploration questions 117, 122, 123
  fatherhood 40–2, 46–8, 108–9
  mind–body connection of
      pregnancy 18, 19, 20, 24
  motherhood 27, 34–8, 46, 107, 117
  postpartum depression 95, 122
  preparing for parenthood 5, 7, 11–
      12
welcoming baby home 73

Yaffe, Sumner 99
Yates, Andrea 90

Zoloft 94, 97, 98, 100